Healthy HORMONES

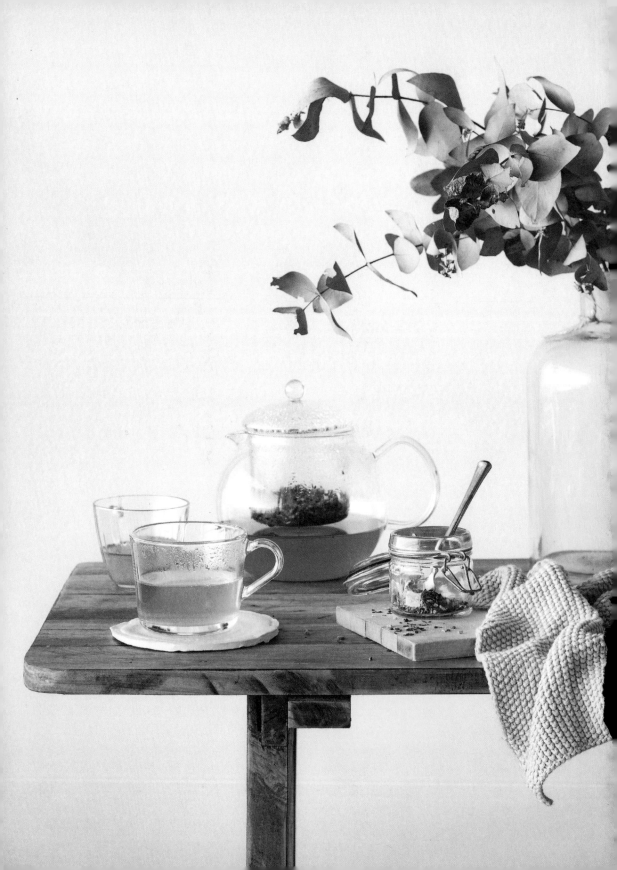

Healthy HORMONES

A PRACTICAL GUIDE TO BALANCING YOUR HORMONES

BELINDA KIRKPATRICK
M.Rep.Med, BHSc(Nat)
& AINSLEY JOHNSTONE

MURDOCH BOOKS
SYDNEY · LONDON

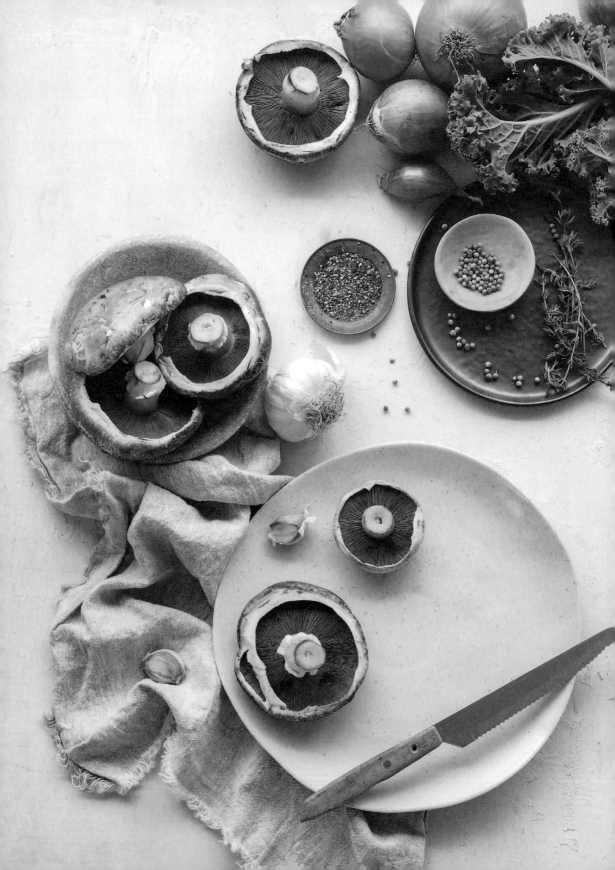

contents

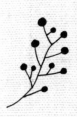

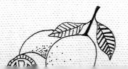

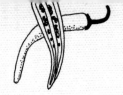

BELINDA KIRKPATRICK (left) is an expert naturopath and nutritionist with both a naturopathic degree and a Master of Reproductive Health. She practises an evidence-based approach to integrative healthcare and offers extensive knowledge of natural and conventional treatments.

Belinda's tertiary qualifications are: Master of Reproductive Health, Bachelor of Health Science (Naturopathy), Associate Diploma in Clinical Sciences and Advanced Diploma of Naturopathy.

Belinda is in clinical practice in Sydney, Australia; is the creator of the Seed iPhone app; is on the expert panel of *Women's Fitness* magazine; designs smoothie and juice recipes for commercial use; is a mother of two beautiful girls; feels like a full-time cook and is a constant time juggler.

AINSLEY JOHNSTONE (right) is a food stylist, recipe developer, illustrator and photographer. Nutritious food is Ainsley's key area of interest. This has come about from working closely with nutritionists, naturopaths and wellbeing experts such as Belinda.

Ainsley has always been creative; this passion began at art school, followed by work in the creative department of an advertising agency, where her skills in art direction, design and typography developed.

Her love of food styling was ignited when she got to work alongside some of the best food stylists in New York. Ever since, she has been working with talented photographers creating imagery for advertising, television, cookbook and editorial clients.

Ainsley is a passionate advocate for mental health and wellbeing. She lives in Sydney with her husband, two daughters and her dog, Cookie.

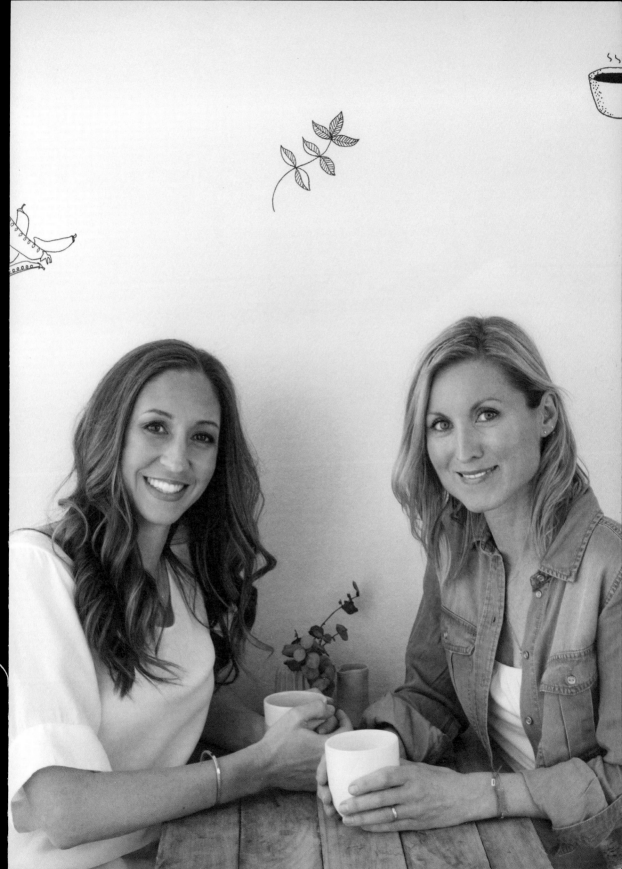

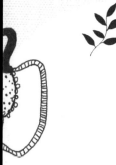

welcome

· ·

This book is a naturopathic and nutritional wealth of information designed for women who want to take an active interest in optimising their hormonal health and understanding more about the ways they can improve their health with good nutrition.

Many health issues experienced by women are affected by hormones. Even if you are not actively trying to conceive or suffering from a specific hormone-related problem, your hormones are still important. If you want to live a healthier and happier life, this book is for you.

Over a decade of clinical experience specialising in women's health has made me passionate about hormonal health, fertility management and miscarriage prevention. My aim is to help women to take charge of their hormones, increase their energy levels, reduce menstrual symptoms or achieve conception. Many women I see in my clinic are confused about what to eat, which supplements to take or at a loss to understand what they can do about unwanted monthly symptoms, difficulty in conceiving or recurrent miscarriage. After identifying the underlying factors using pathology testing and dietary analysis, I use nutritional supplements and herbal medicines along with dietary changes and lifestyle modifications to help women toward better health.

It was during the creation of the Seed period-tracking app (launched in 2016) that I had the opportunity to collaborate with recipe master, food stylist and photographer extraordinaire, Ainsley Johnstone, who created the recipes for this book. Our aim was to ensure that our recipes would be easy to make and not require too many obscure ingredients. Every recipe is designed to support optimal hormonal balance and contains the perfect balance of protein, 'good' fats and something fresh (a mantra that you will soon get to know). The recipes are nutrient-dense, gluten-free, mostly grain-free and with minimal dairy to give you a wide choice for every dietary requirement.

This book is all about gaining knowledge and making choices. It's not necessary to follow all of the advice all of the time in order to be healthy or have healthy hormones: I firmly believe in balance and that making healthy choices most of the time is great. Treats and sweets can be enjoyed without guilt for special celebrations or occasions. Just do what you can or what works for you and try not to stress about things you are not doing. Even small dietary changes or movements toward better health can make a difference, so be proud of yourself and know that your journey towards health is your own and that you don't need to aim for some kind of perfection.

Belinda

belindakirkpatrick.com.au
theseedconcept.com

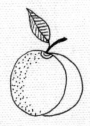

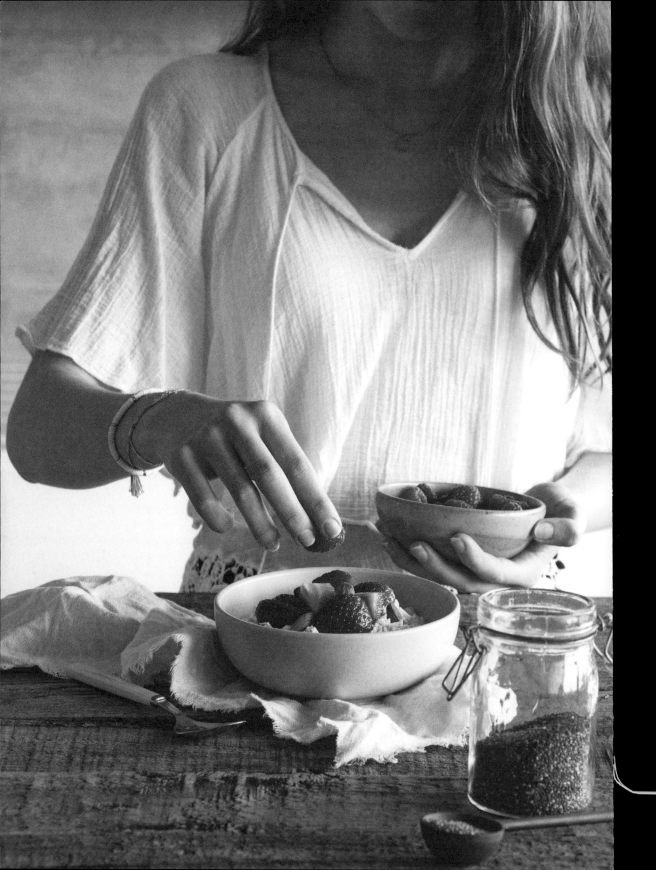

Hormonal Balance

· ·

WHAT IS
hormonal balance?

Hormones are chemical messengers that relay information and instructions to our cells and organs. Hormones give us energy, keep us happy, help us sleep, keep us warm, control hunger and satiety; they regulate our periods, ensure ovulation, control menstrual symptoms, initiate menopause and, of course, contribute to conception and pregnancy.

Hormonal balance refers to the way that these processes promote health and wellbeing. There are more than a hundred hormones that work together to keep us feeling healthy. When the balance of one hormone is disrupted, it impacts on other hormones and can cause ill health.

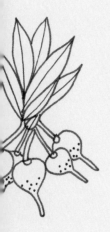

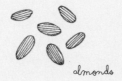

almonds

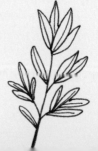

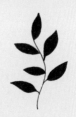

When hormonal balance is optimal, health will be optimal and negative symptoms will be minimal. When hormonal balance is poor, wellbeing may be compromised. The main hormones we will be discussing in this book include oestrogen, progesterone and testosterone, which are the major reproductive hormones; cortisol and adrenaline, the stress hormones; the thyroid hormones, which are responsible for energy and metabolism; and melatonin, our major sleep hormone.

Most women of reproductive age experience hormonal changes on a daily basis. If hormonal balance is compromised, negative symptoms may be experienced throughout the menstrual cycle: these might include period pain, ovulation pain, fluid retention, acne, sugar cravings, digestive disturbances, fatigue, poor mood and much more. This makes hormone production and balance essential for health and happiness.

The most common signs of hormonal imbalance include:

- irregular or absent periods
- painful periods
- irritability or moodiness
- weight gain
- acne
- fatigue
- fertility problems

WHEN HORMONE LEVELS ARE NOT BALANCED, WE DON'T FEEL WELL AND CAN SUFFER FROM A VARIETY OF SYMPTOMS.

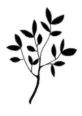

THE MENSTRUAL CYCLE

The menstrual cycle can be broken down into four phases. These include menstruation, the follicular phase, ovulation and the luteal phase.

MENSTRUATION

Menstruation begins on day one of the cycle, the first day of bleeding. When implantation of the fertilised ovum (egg) does not occur, progesterone (and oestrogen) levels drop, which causes the thickened endometrium (lining of the uterus) to break down. The menstrual bleed contains blood, cells from the uterine lining and cervical mucus. Most women wear tampons, pads or menstrual cups during their bleed.

FOLLICULAR PHASE

On day one of the menstrual cycle the pituitary gland in the brain releases follicle stimulating hormone (FSH). This hormone stimulates the ovaries to produce 6–12 tiny follicles, each containing an immature egg. Each cycle, one of these follicles dominates and prepares to release (ovulate) a mature egg while the others die off. Follicle development causes a rise in oestrogen level, which causes the uterine lining to thicken in preparation for a potential pregnancy.

OVULATION

Ovulation generally occurs around two weeks before menstruation. Rising oestrogen from follicle development causes the hypothalamus in the brain to release gonadotropin releasing hormone (GnRH). This stimulates further production of FSH. At a certain level, oestrogen feeds back to the hypothalamus, luteinising hormone (LH) surge occurs and the dominant follicle ovulates. Luteinising hormone is the hormone commonly measured in urinary ovulation test kits. Around 36–48 hours after the surge in LH levels, the egg is released into the fallopian tube and is moved toward the uterus by tiny hairlike projections. It is here in the tube that the egg is either fertilised or will die, usually within 12–24 hours.

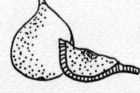

LUTEAL PHASE

The luteal phase refers to the time between ovulation and menstruation and will usually be around 14 days. When the egg is released from its follicle during ovulation, the ruptured follicle remains on the surface of the ovary and becomes the corpus luteum. The corpus luteum releases progesterone, which, along with oestrogen, helps to keep the lining of the uterus thick in preparation for a fertilised egg to implant.

If the egg is fertilised, it may implant into the lining of the uterus and produce hormones to maintain the pregnancy and the corpus luteum, which continues to produce progesterone until the placenta is fully developed and takes over the production of progesterone at around 10 weeks of gestation. Maintaining a healthy pregnancy requires adequate progesterone levels.

If pregnancy has not occurred, the corpus luteum will die and progesterone levels will drop, which causes the uterine lining to stop thickening and begin to shed. The cycle of menstruation begins again.

THE TIME BETWEEN OVULATION AND YOUR PERIOD IS USUALLY 14 DAYS.

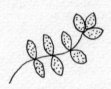

CHOOSE ORGANIC

It is important to consider using organic tampons and pads. Cotton is one of the most heavily sprayed crops and most sanitary items are also bleached in the manufacturing process. Many pesticides, herbicides and bleaches are considered to be hormonal (endocrine) disruptors that can potentially affect health and hormones. The fewer of these substances that we have in our environment, the better.

WHAT IS A NORMAL MENSTRUAL CYCLE?

There is a wide variation in menstrual cycles and it is important to recognise the difference between what is common and what is normal. While period pain is common, many women mistakenly believe that this type of pain is normal, even when it is severe. A menstrual cycle should ideally be free of negative symptoms. Many women will just experience their bleed each month.

LENGTH OF CYCLE

Generally speaking, the average length of a normal menstrual cycle is 28 days, but anywhere from 25–33 days is considered to be within the normal range. A menstrual cycle is calculated by counting from day one, the first full day of bright red bleeding, until the next day one. To get very technical, if you start bleeding in the late afternoon or evening, day one is officially not considered to start until the following day. Spotting is considered to be part of the previous cycle so day one doesn't start until there is actual flow.

FLOW

Normal bleeding will usually last from three to five days and can range from light to moderate or heavy. A flow that is very light (only needing one or two panty liners per day) or super-heavy (flooding or leaking while changing a super pad or tampon every one to two hours) is not normal and should be reported to your GP for investigation. Flow may start off heavy and get progressively lighter or start quite light before becoming heavier, then tapering back to light again. The flow should ideally not start with more than half a day of spotting or end with more than one or two days of spotting (as opposed to light flow).

COLOUR

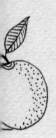

Menstrual flow should be a bright red colour, as though you have just cut yourself, although it may be a deeper darker red when the flow is heavy. There should be minimal to no clotting, although some stringy clots are normal. It is advisable to check with your GP or specialist if you see large or dense clots.

SYMPTOMS

While some women will experience a completely symptom-free menstrual cycle, many women will experience some discomfort. Mild symptoms that do not interfere with your life and only last a day or two before your period are generally considered normal and not an issue, but symptoms that last longer than a few days or disrupt your daily activities are not normal and should be investigated. Common symptoms include nausea, loose stools, headaches, dizziness, fluid retention, fatigue, insomnia, depression, anxiety and irritability, to name a few.

The cause of negative symptoms or premenstrual syndrome (PMS) is not entirely known. Possibilities include hormonal imbalance (oestrogen excess, progesterone deficiency), nutritional deficiencies (particularly vitamin B6 and magnesium), electrolyte imbalances, poor thyroid health, abnormal glucose metabolism and a variety of lifestyle factors. Major lifestyle risk factors for PMS include being overweight, smoking and experiencing high stress. Poor nutrition, dehydration, caffeine and alcohol are also risk factors.

A normal menstrual cycle should be pain free. Unfortunately, many women do experience menstrual pain and cramping, which is known as dysmenorrhoea. Dysmenorrhoea can be classified as primary (from the onset of menstruation) or secondary (due to a physical cause; it usually has a later onset). Women with dysmenorrhoea may suffer painful uterine cramping, back and thigh pain in addition to other symptoms such as nausea, vomiting, diarrhoea, dizziness, fainting and headaches. Dysmenorrhoea can vary in severity from cycle to cycle.

THERE IS A WIDE RANGE OF NORMAL IN AN AVERAGE MENSTRUAL CYCLE AND WHAT IS NORMAL FOR YOU MAY BE DIFFERENT TO WHAT IS NORMAL FOR SOMEBODY ELSE.

SPOTTING BETWEEN PERIODS

Prolonged spotting is often a sign of corpus luteum insufficiency and low progesterone levels. If you are trying to conceive, and experiencing spotting for more than two days before your period, it is a good idea to have your progesterone levels tested with a simple blood test, which can be organised by your GP. This is ideally done one week after ovulation, when progesterone levels should be peaking.

WHEN AM I FERTILE?

Knowing when you are fertile relies on being able to identify when you are ovulating. For most women, this will be around 14 days before your next period is due. This is obviously much easier to calculate for those with a regular cycle and harder to calculate for those with an Irregular cycle. Some women will have what is called a 'luteal phase defect', which means that the time from ovulation to the next period is much shorter than 14 days. This isn't very common, but it can interfere with conception, so it is worth being aware of it if you have been trying to conceive for some time.

In any given month there is generally only a small window of around six days when you are potentially fertile. Learning how to identify your fertile window is super-important for conception but can also be useful for contraceptive purposes. Once you have ovulated, a healthy egg only lasts for 12–24 hours. After this time, you are probably not fertile for the rest of that cycle. Sperm, on the other hand, can survive for three to five days. This means that it is possible to have intercourse five days before ovulation and still conceive. So if the sperm can survive for five days preovulation and the egg can last for one day postovulation, the fertile window is the six days starting from five days before ovulation. Peak fertile time is two days before and the day of ovulation.

Be aware! Some women can ovulate at any part of the cycle. This means that if you are actively trying to avoid conception, you should be very careful and consider a barrier method of contraception throughout the whole month and not just your fertile window.

AM I OVULATING?

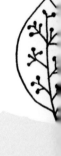

DAY 21 PROGESTERONE

Testing progesterone levels with a blood test is one of the most definitive ways to assess whether you are ovulating. Progesterone levels should be peaking one week past ovulation (which is usually about one week before your period is due). This is easy to pinpoint if you have a regular cycle, but less easy if it is irregular. This test is often called the Day 21 progesterone test but is actually only done on day 21 if you have a 28-day cycle. To calculate when to have your 'Day 21' test, count back seven days from when your period is due and ask a GP or naturopath to test then. For example, if you have a regular 33-day cycle, you would ask your doctor to test progesterone on day 26. While a test result of over 5 nmol/L indicates that you ovulated, your progesterone would ideally be over 30 nmol/L at this time.

TEMPERATURE CHARTING

Charting your basal body temperature can help to pinpoint ovulation and also gives information about what your hormones might be doing at different times of your cycle. Taking your basal body temperature requires you to take your temperature (ideally with a mercury thermometer designed for ovulation testing) as soon as you wake up. This method relies on taking your temperature when you are rested and have had at least four hours of (ideally) uninterrupted sleep. Your temperature must be taken at the same time each morning before you get up, roll over or start chatting, making this quite difficult for people with small children!

Starting on day 1 of your cycle, chart your temperature (see page 22). You should notice that the temperatures are around 36.3°C (97.34°F), rising to around 37°C (98.6°F) in the second half of your cycle. The day that your temperatures dip before they rise is usually when you have ovulated. To know you have ovulated, you must have recorded three consecutive temperatures that are at least 0.1°C (0.2°F) higher than the previous six readings. This method is great for letting you know that you have already ovulated, but doesn't predict in advance when ovulation will occur, making it less useful for timing conception or contraception.

Note: if taking your temperature every day is starting to make you feel anxious and overly focused on every little change, it's time to have a break and switch to an alternative method of assessing ovulation.

OVULATION PREDICTOR KITS

Ovulation predictor kits (OPKs) test urine to help to identify when a woman is fertile by detecting a surge in luteinising hormone (LH), which usually occurs 12–48 hours, but most commonly 24–36 hours, before ovulation. Urine should be tested daily leading up to ovulation until a surge is detected. The LH surge is often best detected in the afternoon around 2pm and urine should be tested at the same time each day. Conception attempts should be regular on the day of the LH surge and the two days following. For some women, particularly those with polycystic ovarian syndrome (PCOS), a positive LH surge may be consistently detected throughout the cycle due to elevated levels of LH. If you are not finding the OPK clear and helpful after two months, try another method of ovulation detection (an unclear OPK result does not necessarily mean you are not ovulating) or see your GP for further investigations.

CERVICAL MUCUS

Why nobody teaches us about cervical mucus when we are learning about periods is beyond me! An understanding of cervical mucus changes can tell you so much about your fertility and is important for both conception and contraception, so it's worth learning about. Cervical mucus is what most women mistakenly identify as discharge. In a regular menstrual cycle, cervical mucus patterns occur at the same time each month. Cervical mucus comes down from the cervix to the mouth of the vagina and is designed to facilitate the passage of sperm into the cervix for conception. The best way to assess cervical mucus is to wait until late in the day (to avoid confusion with residual semen and to wait until the mucus comes down from the cervix to the mouth of the vagina). Wash your hands and, before you do a wee, run two fingers around the mouth of the vagina to see what the mucus feels like.

After your period you will notice that there is not much mucus but that it is sticky. After a week or so, most women will experience a thick white mucus (that looks a bit like moisturising cream) and which some women will notice in their underpants. This type of mucus is thick and sticky and sperm can't swim through it. After this, the mucus

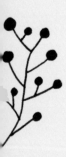

will become more wet, clear and watery under the influence of rising oestrogen levels. This is when you are becoming potentially fertile (for conception and contraception purposes). Sperm can swim through this type of mucus and it makes an easy passage up to the cervix for conception. After a couple of days of this thinner, wetter mucus you may notice a stretchy type of mucus with an eggwhite consistency, which is your peak ovulation type of mucus. Don't worry if you don't see this type of mucus as you may easily miss it. Some women will recognise this type by remembering a time when they used toilet paper to wipe, only to find it quite slippery and needing an extra piece of toilet paper to wipe again. This was probably your most fertile type of mucus and you were most likely ovulating at that time. After this, you may have another day or two of thin and clear mucus before returning to the thick and white or scanty and sticky type of mucus before your period arrives.

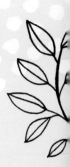

Many women feel strange when they are first learning to test their mucus, but remember that we are all experiencing the same thing every month and the more you learn about your body, the more you can pinpoint ovulation for conception or contraception. Try testing for at least a month or two to learn your own patterns and it will become easier over time.

OVULATION TRACKING

Ovulation tracking is done at a fertility clinic and consists of a series of blood tests and ultrasounds to assess when ovulation is occurring. This process doesn't usually involve a specialist consultation or invasive treatment. Blood tests every two days and ultrasounds allow a thorough assessment of oestrogen, progesterone and luteinising hormone throughout the cycle, allowing ovulation to be anticipated earlier and follicle development confirmed with an ultrasound. Ovulation tracking is useful for people who may not be ovulating at the expected time or need extra help with conception timing.

UNDERSTANDING CERVICAL MUCUS CHANGES CAN TELL YOU SO MUCH ABOUT YOUR FERTILITY AND IS IMPORTANT FOR BOTH CONCEPTION AND CONTRACEPTION, SO IT'S WORTH LEARNING ABOUT.

CHART FOR ONE MENSTRUAL CYCLE

		1	2	3	4	5	6	7	8	9	10	11	12	13	14	15	16	17	18	
DATE																				
DAY OF WEEK																				
DAY OF CYCLE		1	2	3	4	5	6	7	8	9	10	11	12	13	14	15	16	17	18	

TEMPERATURE — Base temperature rises by one box each half hour (usual rising time ___ : ___ hours)

	37.3																			
	37.2																			
	37.1																			
	37.0																			
	36.9																			
	36.8																			
	36.7																			
	36.6																			
	36.5																			
	36.4																			
	36.3																			
	36.2																			
	36.1																			
	36.0																			

CONDITIONS AFFECTING TEMPERATURE

CERVICAL MUCUS																				
	Texture																			
	Colour																			
	Amount																			
	External sensation																			

SECONDARY SYMPTOMS																				
	Pain																			
	Headaches																			
	Nausea																			
	Skin																			
	Breasts																			
	Bowels																			
	Fatigue																			
	Fluid retention																			
	PMS																			

INTERCOURSE																				
BLEEDING																				

		19	20	21	22	23	24	25	26	27	28	29	30	31	32	33	34	35	36	37	38	39	40

COPY
THIS

WHEN SHOULD I SEEK HELP?

Many women choose to seek help from both their GP and a specialist such as a gynaecologist or endocrinologist, in addition to a complementary medicine specialist such as a naturopath, nutritionist or acupuncturist.

Consider seeking help if you:

- Have long, irregular cycles that are more than 33 days in length.

- Have been following the meal plans and lifestyle tips in this book, but have still not had a period in over three months.

- Have regular cycles but do not seem to see a temperature shift, notice mucus changes or get a clear reading on ovulation predictor kits.

- Have been trying to conceive for over six months or are planning on conceiving in the next three months.

- Have very light periods (needing only a panty liner per day).

- Have very heavy periods (leaking, flooding or changing super tampons or pads every one to two hours).

- Experience large clots with menstruation, bigger than 2 cm (¾ inch) diameter.

- Experience pain that requires more than two lots of two painkillers per cycle (or when painkillers do not take your pain away).

- Have premenstrual symptoms that are severe or last longer than three days before your period (including spotting, sore breasts, fluid retention, mood changes, pain, fatigue, bowel changes, bloating, dizziness, headaches, nausea, insomnia or food cravings).

- Experience midcycle pain, which interferes with daily activities.

- Find that your period length or symptoms have changed for the past three months.

A NATUROPATH CAN HELP YOU TO FEEL YOUR BEST, USING HERBAL AND NUTRITIONAL MEDICINE IN ADDITION TO DIETARY AND LIFESTYLE MODIFICATIONS.

WHO CAN HELP ME?

A referral to a specialist gynaecologist or endocrinologist can be helpful in many situations and if you have a hormonal condition it is essential to have a good specialist on your team to investigate any underlying issues or pathology. Be sure to do your research and ask around to ensure that the specialist you are being referred to is a good fit for you. A specialist referral may not be necessary for those with less serious issues.

A naturopath who is also qualified in reproductive medicine will be able to help you make sense of orthodox treatment options, including contraceptives and the huge range of IVF options; give you recommendations for doctors and specialists to consider; and ensure that any supplements you are taking are safe and effective to use alongside your medication.

Reproductive health problems usually arise from a combination of genetic, environmental, inflammatory and immune components. After investigating and treating underlying health problems, by improving diet and lifestyle and implementing appropriate nutritional supplementation with the help of a naturopath many women will achieve a dramatic improvement in their health and symptoms. For those trying to conceive, naturopathy can help many couples achieve their dream of a healthy full-term pregnancy.

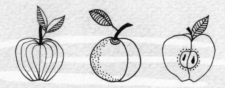

ARE MY HORMONES BALANCED?

Our hormones affect so much of our physical, mental and emotional health that balance is essential. While there are more than a hundred different hormones, we are focusing particularly on the female reproductive hormones where the most common imbalances are found between oestrogen and progesterone. It is these imbalances that cause many of the niggling symptoms that might not necessarily be considered a medical problem, but may impact health and wellbeing on a monthly basis; symptoms such as PMS, moodiness, breast tenderness, pain or fluid retention.

A REPRODUCTIVE HEALTH NATUROPATH CAN HELP YOU TO INTERPRET TEST RESULTS. OPTIMAL HEALTH IS WHAT WE ARE AIMING FOR, NOT JUST ABSENCE OF ILL HEALTH.

Hormone levels fluctuate on a daily basis so, to assess them properly, they should be tested at baseline to allow comparison from month to month. A baseline hormone profile usually includes testing for oestrogen, progesterone, luteinising hormone (LH), follicle stimulating hormone (FSH), prolactin and androgens. Baseline is on day three of the cycle, or on the third day of bleeding. Measuring on this day allows hormone levels to be back at the beginning of the cycle and any hormonal hangover from the previous cycle should have been cleared. Progesterone should be low at this time and should also be tested one week after ovulation (or one week before the period is due), as that is when it should be peaking. Measuring both levels will allow a full assessment of hormonal health. It is worth noting that hormones can be difficult to test and blood or saliva testing just provides a snapshot for direction; it does not measure levels of environmental oestrogens, which are hormone-like compounds that are absorbed into the body and can create unwanted oestrogen-like effects. The reference range for the hormones is wide, so falling within the range of normal does not necessarily mean that your hormones are balanced or at optimal levels. A reproductive health naturopath can help you to interpret your test results. Optimal health is what we are aiming for, not just absence of ill health.

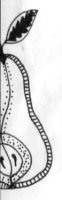

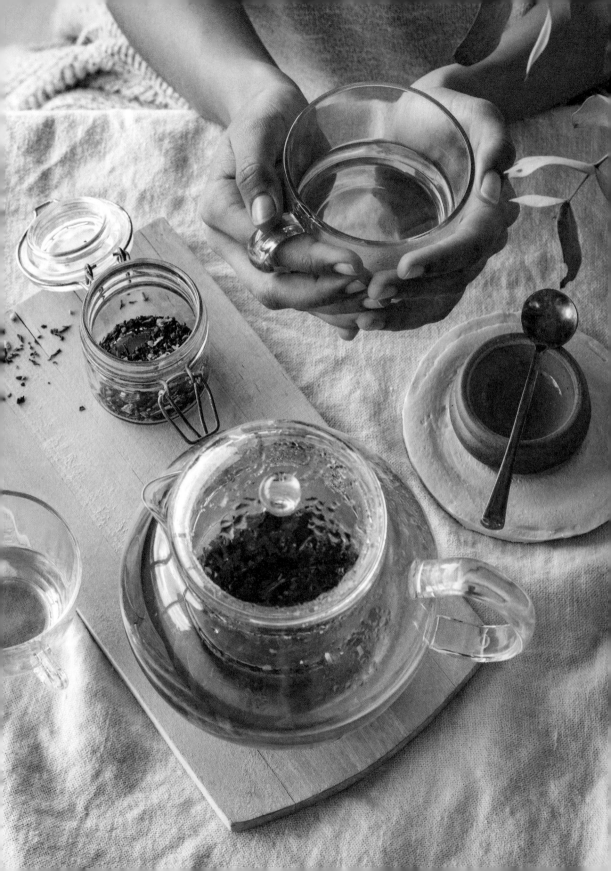

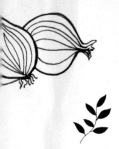

RELATIVE OESTROGEN EXCESS

Oestrogen excess is not usually caused by an overproduction of oestrogen by the ovaries, but is more likely to be due to lifestyle factors, such as environmental oestrogens, dietary choices, poor clearance of oestrogen from the body, obesity or inadequate levels of progesterone. It is not always a true excess of oestrogen, but sometimes it is an excess relative to the levels of other hormones.

Oestrogen exposure has increased in modern times due, in part, to lifestyle choices. Compared to our grandparents' time, women today tend to have fewer pregnancies, spend less time breastfeeding, and have an earlier onset of menarche (the first period) and a later age of menopause. This means that we tend to have more menstrual cycles and therefore more natural oestrogen over our lifetimes. It's possible that this exposure contributes to the onset of oestrogen-dependent conditions such as endometriosis (when the uterine lining grows outside the uterus), breast cancer, fibroids (benign tumours in the uterus) and adenomyosis (when lining tissue grows inside the muscular walls of the uterus).

WHAT ARE ENVIRONMENTAL OESTROGENS?

Environmental oestrogens are a group of more than 800 chemicals also known as endocrine disrupting chemicals (EDCs) or xenoestrogens. These chemicals are thought to affect hormonal balance[1] and can interfere with reproductive health and fetal development. They are found in everyday products such as cleaning chemicals, handwash, fragrant candles, pesticides used on conventional produce, perfumes, make-up, nail polish and many more. Plastics (even BPA-free plastic) may release these chemicals, particularly when heated and cooled. Learn more about what to avoid on pages 88–93 and start minimising your exposure to these products today by slowly switching over to natural alternatives.

Poor clearance of oestrogen

Oestrogen is mostly metabolised and removed from the body via the liver, bowels and kidneys. Adequate clearance of oestrogen is essential for hormone balance. If the bowels are sluggish or liver and kidney function is not optimal, oestrogen clearance is reduced. Look after these organs by minimising alcohol and caffeine, drinking plenty of filtered water and prioritising your diet to improve bowel function: increase vegetable and dietary fibre intake, reduce saturated fats (especially from conventionally farmed sources), increase gut-loving fermented foods (that foster the growth of 'good' bacteria) such as sauerkraut, kimchi, kefir and miso, as well as getting regular exercise.

Why your weight matters

Obesity can interfere with ovulation and hormonal balance. Too much fatty tissue increases the conversion of androgens (hormones such as testosterone) to oestrogen, which creates a relative excess and increases the risk factors for many oestrogen-dependent conditions. Increasing exercise and focusing on a nutritious diet containing adequate protein and an abundance of vegetables is often the first step in managing this problem. Concurrent hormonal conditions experienced by many obese women—including polycystic ovarian syndrome (PCOS)—can make weight loss difficult and frustrating. Your naturopath or GP can offer individual guidance, motivation and support.

Low progesterone

Another cause of oestrogen excess is when levels of progesterone are inadequate. Progesterone balances the effects of oestrogen and reduces the risk of oestrogen-dependent medical conditions. Oestrogen is completely unopposed by progesterone when women are not ovulating, but may be inadequately opposed when progesterone levels are low due to stress, poor diet or nutritional deficiencies.

Common symptoms of oestrogen excess

- Mood swings
- Uterine fibroids
- Irritability
- Facial flushing
- Fluid retention
- Heavy periods
- Period pain
- Fatigue
- Sugar cravings
- Easy weight gain

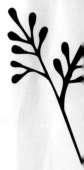

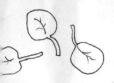

PRACTICAL TIPS TO REDUCE OESTROGEN EXCESS

Eat two to three cups of broccoli, cauliflower, asparagus, fennel, kale, spinach and brussels sprouts most days. Brassica vegetables contain substances that help to conjugate and remove excess oestrogen from the body via the liver.

Avoid using plastic food wrap and plastic water bottles and heating food in plastic containers. These are major sources of environmental oestrogens. Glass containers can be used instead.

Detoxify from environmental oestrogen by following the recommendations in the Lifestyle section (see page 86).

To reduce inflammation in the gut, consider trying to avoid dairy, gluten, corn, soy and sugar.

Decrease red meat to around one serve per week (but increase organically produced chicken and eggs and sustainably caught fish).

Eat organically produced foods to decrease levels of oestrogen exposure. Check out your local farmers' markets for low-toxin options that are not too expensive.

Add 1–2 tablespoons of freshly ground linseeds (flaxseeds) to food or drinks daily. Linseeds contain lignan, which is believed to help eliminate excess oestrogen from your system. High intake of lignan is not recommended if you are pregnant or breastfeeding.

Also aim to drink two to three cups of liver-friendly herbal teas most days. These include nettle, dandelion root or leaf, globe artichoke and St Mary's thistle (milk thistle).

Stay well hydrated. I recommend at least 1.5 litres (52 fl oz/6 cups) of water per day, aiming for your urine to be a light colour.

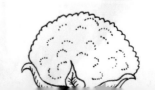

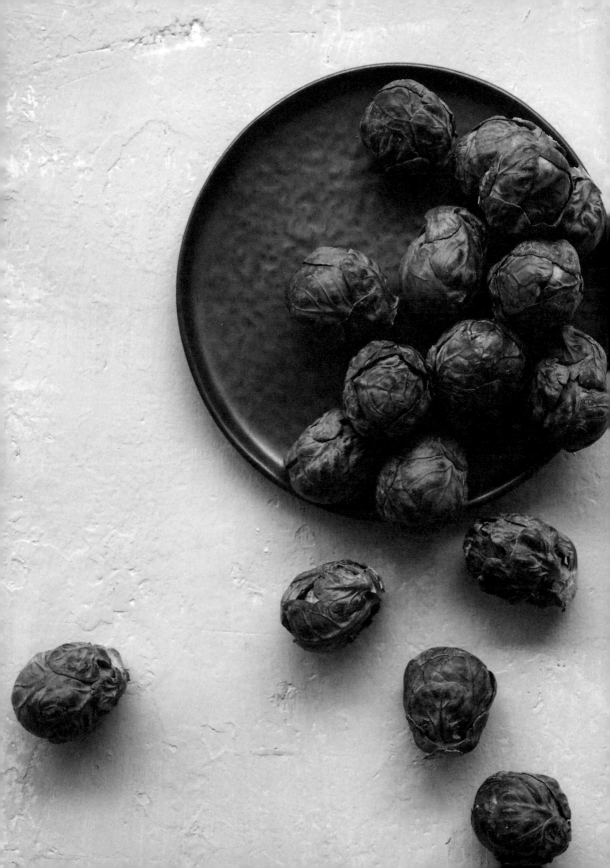

RELATIVE OESTROGEN DEFICIENCY

Low oestrogen can be just as much of a problem as high oestrogen. Oestrogen deficiency (confirmed by a blood test) often occurs when body weight is very low, which results in a lower conversion rate of androgens to oestrogen. It may be exacerbated when bowel movements occur very frequently and when fibre intake is too high and available oestrogen is bound up and excreted from the body. True oestrogen deficiency occurs after menopause, when ovarian reserve is very low, or when the ovaries are removed.

Low body weight (or low body fat) is a common cause of low oestrogen that can interrupt the menstrual cycle and make it erratic or absent. This is an issue, because both bone density and fertility may be impacted. Excessive exercise (with or without low body weight) can also reduce the level of oestrogen. If your cycle is absent or irregular and you do high-intensity cardio exercise more than twice a week, reduce the cardio exercise and replace it with walking, yoga and gentle strength-based exercises.

Dietary fibre is known to increase oestrogen clearance and reduce circulating oestrogen levels. This is great when everything is balanced, but when too much is excreted it is not available for use in the body. Excess fibre can cause multiple loose bowel movements daily. It is really about making sure your diet is balanced: moderation is the key.

Common symptoms of oestrogen deficiency

- Poor memory
- Candida (thrush) infections
- Night sweats
- Dry skin
- Long or irregular menstrual cycles

- Palpitations
- Depression
- Insomnia
- Low libido
- Vaginal dryness

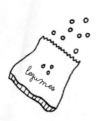

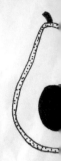

PRACTICAL TIPS

Boost oestrogen levels by adding lots of sesame seeds (such as unhulled tahini), chickpeas and legumes into your diet. These foods contain phytoestrogens that bind to oestrogen receptors and exert an oestrogen-like effect.

....

Increase your intake of red meat (preferably organically farmed or grass-fed) to three times weekly, to increase iron levels.

....

Eat protein with every meal: animal proteins are ideal for supporting regular menstrual cycles and improving mood, focus and sleep. Try frittatas, chicken salads, salmon patties and slow-cooked lamb.

....

Exercise gently two to three days per week. Too much exercise can supress the hypothalamus and reduce oestrogen levels, leading to irregular periods, scanty bleeding, poor moods and low energy levels. Try more gentle forms of exercise such as long walks, yoga and stretching.

....

Aim to gain weight if you are underweight or have low body-fat percentage: do this the healthy way by eating nutritious food regularly and adding nutrient-dense meals and snacks, including starchy foods such as banana, sweet potato and pumpkin.

....

Increase 'good' fats and minimise the 'bad' ones. Fats are essential in a balanced diet. 'Good' fats are found in unheated olive oil, coconut oil, avocado, nuts, seeds, hummus, tahini, oily fish such as tuna and salmon. 'Bad' fats are found in processed oils, fried foods, margarine, processed biscuits and popcorn and anything containing canola or sunflower oil.

....

Avoid soy products. Despite the ability of soy to boost oestrogen, it is also a nutrient blocker that decreases the absorption of important nutrients and minerals. It can also inhibit thyroid function and is heavily processed. Fermented forms of soy, such as miso, tempeh and tamari, are fine in moderation.

....

Up your vegetable intake. Aim for seven-plus types every day. Foods that help boost oestrogen include apples, alfalfa, cherries, chickpeas (garbanzo beans), carrots, celery, cucumbers, dates, fennel, olive oil, papaya, peas, plums, pomegranates, potatoes, legumes, rhubarb and tomatoes.

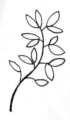

PROGESTERONE DEFICIENCY

Progesterone is produced from the corpus luteum after ovulation (or by the placenta in pregnancy). Progesterone deficiency can be caused by: failure to ovulate and ovulation disorders, abnormal follicle development, luteal phase defects, thyroid issues or high stress levels. Conditions commonly associated with lack of progesterone include polycystic ovarian syndrome (PCOS), hypothalamic amenorrhoea, dysfunctional uterine bleeding and hyperprolactinaemia. If you suspect you are not ovulating, see your GP for investigations and diagnosis.

When ovulation doesn't occur, less progesterone is produced, which means that underlying conditions must be addressed before ovulation and progesterone production can resume. Abnormal follicle development or luteinisation, seen when levels of follicle stimulating hormone (FSH) and luteinising hormone (LH) are too low, can also contribute to decreased progesterone production from poor ovulation.

An inadequate luteal phase or 'luteal phase defect' is when the lining of the uterus does not thicken properly each month. This can occur when the ovaries do not release enough progesterone or the lining of the uterus doesn't respond properly to the progesterone, resulting in a shortened luteal phase of around 10 days, and may result in spotting, miscarriage or difficulty conceiving. The ideal luteal phase is around 14 days.

Thyroid hormones stimulate the release of progesterone in the second half of a woman's cycle, making a healthy thyroid essential to a healthy cycle. Many women suffer from suboptimal thyroid function despite being told that their thyroid is normal. Suboptimal or subclinical hypothyroidism can lower progesterone, lengthening your cycle and negatively affecting conception and pregnancy maintenance. To fully assess thyroid function, a test can be done by your GP. The range for thyroid stimulating hormone (TSH) is usually 0.4–4.5 mIU/L, and should be under 2.5 mIU/L for women who are trying to conceive.

Common symptoms of progesterone deficiency

- Enlarged breasts
- Breakthrough bleeding
- Low libido
- Short menstrual cycles
- PMS
- Spotting
- Headaches
- Anxiety
- Cramping pain
- Early miscarriage

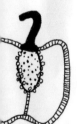

PRACTICAL TIPS

Reducing stress is one of the most important things you can do to support progesterone production. Spend a few minutes every day doing this simple exercise: sit comfortably and take 10 deep, slow breaths. Hold each breath for a few seconds at the peak of the inhale and exhale. This simple technique switches on the parasympathetic nervous system while switching off that stressful fight-or-flight mode that most of us function in on a regular basis.

....

Learn to say no and stop overcommitting yourself.

....

Take a relaxing and detoxifying bath by adding one cup of Epsom salts (magnesium sulphate) to the water. Do this for at least 15 minutes twice weekly to relax and allow the magnesium from the salts to absorb through the skin.

....

Prioritise getting enough sleep (seven to nine hours is recommended for most people) every night.

....

Implement a regular yoga, mindfulness or meditation practice. You don't have to be good at it, you just have to try.

....

Consider a supplement containing magnesium and vitamin B6: these nutrients are essential for progesterone production and can help to reduce PMS, regulate menstruation and boost mood. Foods rich in these nutrients include chicken, turkey, silverbeet (Swiss chard), sunflower seeds and pistachio nuts.

....

Increase your vitamin C intake, which can restore the adrenal glands and support hormone balance. Eat at least two to three serves of vitamin C-rich foods most days; try papaya, capsicum (pepper), broccoli, Brussels sprouts, strawberries, pineapple, oranges, kiwifruit and cauliflower.

....

Vitamin D is a hormone precursor that is essential for progesterone production: with many of us working indoors or being super-sunsmart, vitamin D levels are often low. You can have your vitamin D levels tested by your GP.

STRESS AND CONCEPTION

Progesterone is essential for a healthy luteal phase and a successful pregnancy but when your body is producing lots of stress hormones, progesterone levels drop. When you are stressed, your adrenal glands produce the stress hormones cortisol and adrenaline. To make cortisol, however, your adrenal glands need progesterone and when cortisol is needed, progesterone will always be used, no matter how little you already have available. When you are chronically stressed (or even, like many of us, chronically busy and running on cortisol and adrenaline) progesterone levels become low. Reducing stress, and restoring healthy adrenal function, may improve progesterone levels.[2]

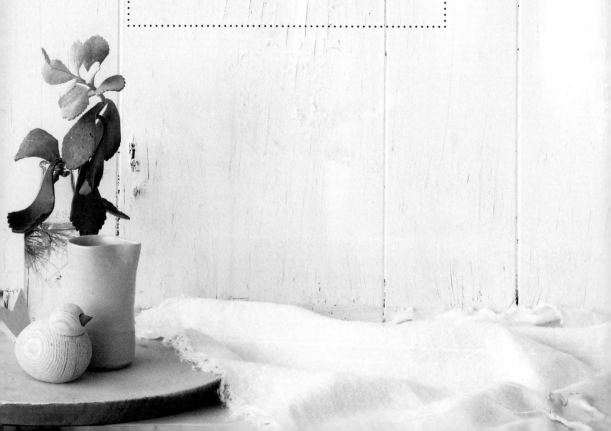

PERIOD PAIN

PRIMARY DYSMENORRHOEA

Primary dysmenorrhoea, also known simply as period pain, is defined as painful menstruation that occurs in the absence of underlying pathology such as endometriosis and ovarian cysts. Primary dysmenorrhoea will usually start on day one of menstrual flow and last for two to three days. The pain is most often cramping in the lower abdomen that may radiate to the lower back or thighs.

Prostaglandins

Primary dysmenorrhoea is often due to a prostaglandin imbalance. Prostaglandins are hormone-like substances that cause inflammation, blood vessel constriction, blood clotting, muscle contractions and pain. Prostaglandins in the uterus are required to help the uterine muscles to contract and shed the lining during menstruation. Severe contractions can restrict the blood vessels and deprive the uterine muscles of oxygen, leading to further pain. Lots of prostaglandins means lots of pain.

Prostaglandins can also enter the bloodstream and contribute to other symptoms such as diarrhoea, nausea and headaches. Nonsteroidal anti-inflammatory medication, such as ibuprofen (also known as Nurofen, Advil and Motrin), works by decreasing prostaglandin production, therefore reducing the level of pain. Luckily, there are several dietary and lifestyle modifications and nutritional supplements (including fish oils and turmeric) that can also help to mediate prostaglandin release.

Endorphins

Beta-endorphins are produced by the body to provide an analgesic (pain relieving) effect, in addition to increasing the rate of prostaglandin breakdown and thus reducing pain and cramping. A lack of beta-endorphins can also contribute to excessive pain. Beta-endorphins are released during aerobic or cardio exercise and are known as internal opioids or natural pain relievers.

BETA-ENDORPHINS ARE RELEASED DURING AEROBIC OR CARDIO EXERCISE AND ARE KNOWN AS INTERNAL OPIOIDS OR NATURAL PAIN RELIEVERS.

Inflammation

A certain level of inflammation is a normal part of the menstrual cycle. Inflammatory prostaglandins, made from omega-6 fatty acids, trigger both ovulation and menstruation. Chronic or excessive inflammation, however, can result in menstrual pain and cramping and disrupted ovulation. Omega-3 fatty acids can help to increase the production of anti-inflammatory prostaglandins. A diet high in fresh vegetables and low in processed food, and the use of supplements, such as fish oils and turmeric, recommended by a naturopath, can significantly reduce inflammation and reduce period pain. The Mediterranean diet, which includes lots of vegetables, fruits, nuts, fish and 'good' oils and contains minimal processed foods, is great for supplying omega-3 fatty acids.[3]

Risk factors

Risk of menstrual cramps and pain is increased in women who:

- Started to menstruate before age 11

- Have heavy periods

- Have irregular cycles

- Have never given birth

- Are smokers

- Have a family history of painful periods

- Have an underlying medical condition (see opposite)

If your menstrual cramping and pain disrupts your life or is progressively worsening, you should see your healthcare provider. This is really important as so many women believe pain to be normal and live for many years with severe pain or undiagnosed endometriosis that can negatively affect their life and may contribute to longlasting fertility issues.

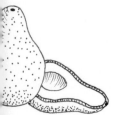

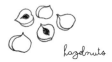

hazelnuts

SECONDARY DYSMENORRHOEA

Secondary dysmenorrhoea is defined as menstrual pain arising from pelvic pathology or an underlying medical condition. The pain is caused by a disease or abnormality in the female reproductive system, including the uterus, ovaries or fallopian tubes. The pain is very similar to menstrual cramping but often lasts longer than the period, starts before it or also occurs at other times of the month. Treating secondary dysmenorrhoea involves identifying and treating the cause, often in conjunction with medical or surgical intervention.

The most common causes include:

- **Endometriosis:** tissue from the uterine lining embedding outside the uterus.

- **Adenomyosis:** benign growths in the uterine walls.

- **Adhesions:** scarring or adherence of two surfaces or structures.

- **Uterine fibroids:** benign growths in or outside the uterus.

- **Pelvic inflammatory disease:** infection of the reproductive organs.

- **Cervical stenosis:** narrowing or closure of the cervix.

- Sexually transmitted diseases

- Copper IUDs

- Ovarian cysts

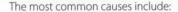

REDUCING STRESS IS ONE OF THE MOST IMPORTANT THINGS YOU CAN DO TO SUPPORT PROGESTERONE PRODUCTION: SPEND A FEW MINUTES EVERY DAY DOING SIMPLE RELAXATION EXERCISES.

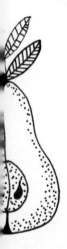

Simple tips
FOR DEALING WITH COMMON SYMPTOMS

Remember that these symptoms may be common but should not be considered normal: it *is* possible to have a symptom-free cycle. If you are experiencing multiple symptoms and are unsure whether they are linked to your cycle, or you simply want to track your progress, you may find it helpful to fill out a menstrual symptom chart such as the one on page 56. Start filling it in on day one of your cycle.

Use the simple nutritional and lifestyle tips in the following pages and learn why certain symptoms might be occurring. These are general recommendations, so if you don't notice an improvement, please see your naturopath for individualised advice before using herbal medicines or nutritional supplements. Be sure to discuss any supplements you are taking with your GP if you are taking any prescription medications.

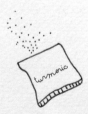

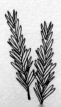

ACNE

Acne and skin breakouts are a nightmare, particularly when they appear after the teenage years. Acne may be caused by a specific bacteria called *Propionibacterium acnes*, nutrient deficiencies, inflammation, or hormonal factors such an androgen excess. Women with high levels of androgens in the bloodstream or very sensitive androgen receptors have increased oil production that can lead to clogged pores and breakouts. Acne breakouts caused by hormones are usually on the lower face, jawline and neck and will often flare up just before or during your period or ovulation. Many doctors will treat acne by prescribing the oral contraceptive pill that contains both oestrogen and progesterone and lowers the amount of androgens that your body produces. Clear skin is one reason for many women going onto or remaining on the Pill; however, it is usually a short-term treatment option. Try the tips below to improve your skin naturally.

TIPS Avoid dairy products as they can cause your skin to produce more oil and clog your pores. Cow's milk is also high in a hormone called insulin-like growth factor 1 (IGF-1), which is great for helping baby calves to grow but can cause inflammation in humans. Many people find that when they give up dairy, acne improves, so try a dairy-free diet for at least a month and assess your skin. Be aware that many dairy replacements contain ingredients such as sunflower oil or sugar, so look for a pure almond or coconut milk as cow's milk replacements. If you decide to avoid dairy in the long term, please see the information about calcium (page 232) to ensure you are getting enough calcium in your daily diet, or if you are considering supplementation.

Reducing inflammation and improving the clearance of hormones by the liver is also essential. Make an extra effort to avoid food and drink containing added sugars and try adding a teaspoon of ground turmeric (known for its anti-inflammatory properties) to your food daily. Ensure good digestive health to keep your gut bacteria in balance by adding a teaspoon of apple cider vinegar to water before meals; you could also take a probiotic supplement before breakfast each day. Ensure you are eating at least five cups of fresh vegetables every day and avoid all fried foods and vegetable oils. See a naturopath for further advice on supplements you can take. If you don't see an improvement in your skin, consult your GP or a naturopath for further advice.

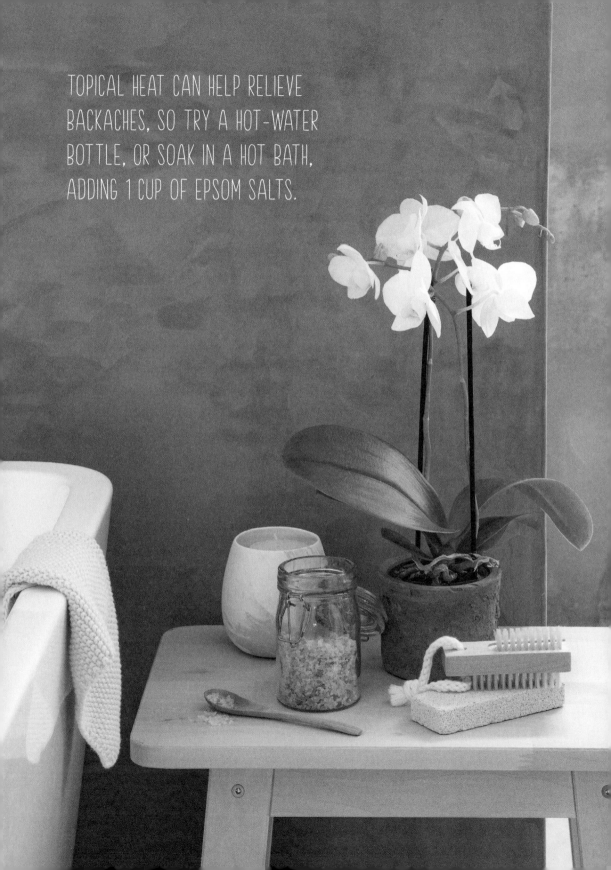

TOPICAL HEAT CAN HELP RELIEVE
BACKACHES, SO TRY A HOT-WATER
BOTTLE, OR SOAK IN A HOT BATH,
ADDING 1 CUP OF EPSOM SALTS.

BACKACHES

Period-related backaches are usually due to the cramping of your uterus, but they can also be caused by a pre-existing structural back problem or endometriosis. As the uterus prepares for menstruation, it produces the hormone-like prostaglandins that cause uterine contractions. When excessive amounts of inflammatory prostaglandins are released, they can cause intense cramping in not only the uterus but also in the lower back and upper thighs and generalised inflammation in the lower abdominal and back area that may aggravate an existing weakness or injury.

TIPS Increase your intake of anti-inflammatory foods such as oily fish, leafy greens, avocado, lemon, pomegranate and almonds. Add freshly grated ginger and turmeric to your food for anti-inflammatory action. Topical heat can help, so try a hot-water bottle, or soak in a hot bath, adding 1 cup of Epsom salts (magnesium sulphate) for best results. Ginger and cinnamon tea can help: try to drink two cups a day while you are having the symptoms. See your GP, physiotherapist or a naturopath if you need further help with back pain.

BLOATING

The general inflammation caused by prostaglandins circulating in the bloodstream can also affect digestion. When the digestive system is inflamed, it is more difficult to break down and absorb the nutrients found in food and as a result further inflammation occurs. During this time (and also during times of illness or convalescence), our digestive systems benefit from well-cooked foods, which are already broken down and do not require too much digestive energy to be absorbed.

TIPS Eat slowly, chew well and include foods that are well-cooked, soaked, stewed, steamed or sprouted; for example, soups, stews, casseroles, stewed or soft fruits, nut pastes, porridges and steamed vegetables. Also include herbs and spices such as ginger, cloves, basil, rosemary, fennel, dill, anise, caraway, cardamom, cumin and parsley. Herbal teas are great between and after meals: fennel, licorice, nettle, peppermint, ginger and chamomile may help reduce bloating. Foods to avoid at this time of the cycle (but which are part of a nutritious diet when digestive function is optimal) include: salads (especially uncooked leaves), hard and raw fruits (particularly apples), whole nuts and undercooked vegetables.

BREAST TENDERNESS

Cyclical breast tenderness and swelling is a common symptom leading up to menstruation. Some women will notice tenderness immediately following ovulation and not get any relief until their period has begun. Cyclical breast tenderness is generally caused by oestrogen dominance or progesterone deficiency. Excess or unopposed oestrogen is inflammatory and causes breast tissue to grow and become tender. Treatments are usually based on reducing excess oestrogen and supporting adequate progesterone production.

TIPS Support your liver in detoxification and oestrogen clearance by avoiding all caffeine and minimising alcohol intake. Try a daily liver-cleansing tea containing herbs such as St Mary's thistle, globe artichoke (jerusalem artichoke) and dandelion root. Reduce inflammation by avoiding 'bad' fats such as vegetable oil, fried foods and margarine. Try adding two tablespoons of freshly ground linseeds (flaxseeds) to your daily diet and make sure you eat plenty of fibre: try to ensure you have at least one bowel movement each day. A naturopath can help with digestive issues.

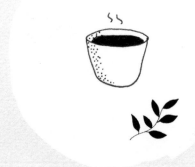

CHOCOLATE CRAVINGS

For years, researchers have debated why so many women crave chocolate just before they get their period and they don't seem to have come up with an answer. Studies have been done on women from a variety of cultures and in different stages of their lives (menstruating, pregnant and postmenopausal) and found little difference in their cravings, leading many to believe that it is the social acceptance of period-related chocolate cravings that causes women to allow themselves chocolate at this time.

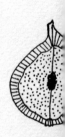

While this may be true for some, after working with thousands of women over the past decade, I can't agree that this theory holds true for everyone. Many women in my clinic don't even think of chocolate all month until their cravings are the first sign that their period is approaching. It seems to me that any or all of the following could potentially be linked to the cravings: magnesium deficiency, blood-sugar fluctuations, hormonal changes or a premenstrual drop in the feel-good neurotransmitter serotonin. Studies so far have not definitively shown these links, but they cannot be ruled out.

TIPS The following ideas have reduced chocolate cravings for many of my clients. Blood-sugar levels are less stable before your period, so avoid sugar and eat regular protein-containing meals and snacks throughout the day: plan your snacks and do not skip a meal. Ensure you are drinking plenty of filtered water and load up on foods such as seeds, dark leafy greens, figs, avocados, fish and lentils that contain higher levels of magnesium. Try a Bliss ball (see page 204). Try to get gentle exercise outside most days. See a naturopath if cravings continue to be a problem.

ENSURE YOU ARE DRINKING PLENTY OF FILTERED WATER AND LOAD UP ON FOODS SUCH AS SEEDS, LEAFY GREENS, FIGS, AVOCADOS, FISH AND LENTILS.

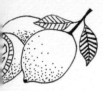

CONSTIPATION

The week before your period is due, increasing progesterone levels can contribute to sluggish bowels or constipation. Progesterone is a muscle relaxant and generally slows digestive function, which can make bowel movements more difficult.

TIPS If this is an issue for you, there are a few things you can do to try to get things moving. Many women don't like going to the toilet at work and hold on to their bowel movements to avoid it. Set an alarm to get up early enough in the morning to start the day with 1 tablespoon of lemon juice in a cup of warm water. After breakfast, make some time to just sit on the toilet (no straining) and allow your bowels time to move.

Increase your regular daily intake of filtered water to about 2 litres (70 fl oz/8 cups). For a bedtime drink, mix 2 tablespoons of chia seeds and 50 ml (1¾ fl oz) of prune juice into 100 ml (3½ fl oz) of water and stir for 5 minutes. Set it aside for a further 10 minutes until a soft gel is formed. Chia seeds contain a soluble form of fibre and are very gentle on the digestive system. Soaking them before consuming ensures that they do not absorb more water in the bowel and worsen constipation. Ensure that your diet is full of cooked vegetables.

These tips can either be followed for the whole month or just the week before your period is due if that is the only time you suffer symptoms of constipation. If constipation is an ongoing problem for you, consult your GP or a naturopath.

HAPPY TUMMY YOGA POSE

Lie on your back with both legs extended straight. Bring your right knee in to your chest and hold it there with both hands. Stay in that pose for 20 deep, slow breaths. Slowly return to your starting position, then reach your right arm up behind you to completely stretch out your right side along the floor. Hold for 10 breaths and then repeat on your left side.

CRAMPS

In the absence of hormonal conditions such as endometriosis, cramping pain is usually caused by the release of excessive prostaglandins, constricted blood flow, oestrogen dominance and inflammation. Cramps can also be caused by constipation. Cramping pain experienced before menstruation or at other times during the cycle should always be investigated by a medical professional, as should pain that is getting worse or interferes with your daily activities.

FOCUS ON DAILY AND ABUNDANT INTAKE OF LIVER-FRIENDLY, OESTROGEN-METABOLISING VEGGIES SUCH AS BROCCOLI, CAULIFLOWER, CABBAGE, KALE, SPINACH AND ASPARAGUS.

TIPS If cramping pain is something that is a part of your monthly cycle, try following these tips for three months and monitor your progress. Reduce inflammation and oestrogen dominance by increasing fibre and fresh vegetables in your diet. Focus on daily and abundant intake of the liver-friendly, oestrogen-metabolising veggies such as broccoli, cauliflower, brussels sprouts, cabbage, kale, spinach and asparagus. Reduce red meat intake to once a week and focus on fish, legumes and organic chicken instead. Try to avoid dairy, sugar, caffeine and processed grains such as white rice and bread that might increase inflammation. These dietary modifications are not easy, but if they help to improve your symptoms they will be worth the trouble. Use the recipes and meal plans in this book for inspiration.

Iodine deficiency is common and iodine is important for oestrogen metabolism. A naturopath can test your levels and recommend iodine supplements if they are necessary.

Detoxify your home from hormone disruptors found in plastics, skin-care products and so on: see the Lifestyle section on page 86 for more details.

When you have cramping period pain, try placing a hot-water bottle on your tummy or have a soak in a hot bath, adding a cup of Epsom salts (magnesium sulphate).

DIARRHOEA

After the premenstrual sluggish bowels associated with progesterone, you might have the opposite problem when your period arrives. Loose bowel movements and stomach cramps can be due to a drop in progesterone levels and the impact of prostaglandin release, which is designed to make the uterus contract, but can also impact the bowels. If your digestion has been really sluggish, the release associated with your period can be a blessing.

TIPS You can dissolve a teaspoon of slippery elm powder in warm water and drink twice daily to ease stomach cramps and loose stools. Eat foods that are not too fibrous and are easy to digest. Avoid foods that are high in fat and sugar. Try a porridge or chia pudding for breakfast and focus on soups and casseroles for lunch and dinner. Exercise very gently at this time. If you have ongoing problems with bowel movements, see your GP to check the cause.

DIZZINESS

Feeling dizzy or lightheaded just before or during menstruation is very common. It is particularly common in women who have low blood pressure or a low pulse rate. There are a few things that may contribute to this, including iron deficiency, heavy bleeding and hypoglycaemia.

Iron deficiency is quite common in menstruating women. Heavy bleeding contributes to iron deficiency. Women with anaemia or very low iron will often suffer from dizziness, blurred vision, fatigue and even vertigo with their periods. Your GP can organise a blood test to check your iron levels and determine if a supplement is necessary. A naturopath can recommend a supplement that won't cause constipation. Too much iron is not a good thing, so always get your iron levels tested before starting any supplementation.

Blood-sugar levels can be variable around the time of menstruation and this might contribute to extreme hunger, sugar cravings and an increased risk of hypoglycaemia. This is when your blood-sugar levels fall too low and you start to feel faint, irritable, tired and dizzy.

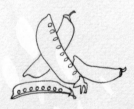

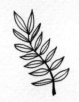

FATIGUE

Fatigue and lethargy are common menstrual symptoms. Energy usually starts to return a few days after your period begins. Fatigue lasting more than a few days may be due to iron deficiency, pain, a sluggish thyroid or high stress levels. Pain can cause fatigue, particularly when it affects your ability to have a good night's sleep. Poor thyroid function or excessive stress and adrenal fatigue are also possibilities. Check ongoing symptoms of fatigue with your GP or naturopath.

TIPS Increase nutritious foods that support oestrogen, such as linseeds (flaxseeds), sesame seeds, chickpeas (garbanzo beans), green peas, alfalfa sprouts and edamame (fresh soya beans). Increase your intake of red meat to three times a week and avoid sugar and caffeine. Drink at least 1.5 litres (52 fl oz/6 cups) or more of filtered water daily, and include two cups of licorice tea per day to combat stress and support adrenal gland function. (Caution: licorice tea can cause or exacerbate high blood pressure.)

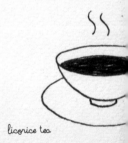

licorice tea

FLUID RETENTION

Fluid retention usually starts in the premenstrual phase of the cycle and peaks in the follicular phase when oestrogen levels are high. In the luteal phase, oestrogen decreases while progesterone increases, which can result in excess fluid in the feet, legs and abdomen. Some women don't clear this fluid easily and find that they end up with fluid retention for much of their cycle. Dehydration and eating too many processed foods can also contribute to fluid retention.

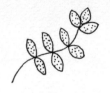

> **TIPS** Drink two to three cups of nettle tea daily to help reduce fluid retention. Avoid salty and processed foods. Potassium can help fluid balance, so be sure to include potassium-rich foods such as bananas, tomatoes, apples and apricots in your diet. Limit your caffeine intake to one cup of tea or coffee daily and continue your regular exercise.

HEADACHES

Premenstrual headaches can occur when oestrogen and progesterone drop to their lowest levels just before and during the first day of menstruation. Higher levels of prostaglandins and lower levels of the body's natural painkilling endorphins may also be responsible. Others will find that their headaches are worse at ovulation, when the liver is struggling to metabolise high oestrogen levels.

Supporting hormonal balance, decreasing inflammation, avoiding headache triggers and supporting liver detoxification are the main aims of treatment.

> **TIPS** Try eliminating gluten, reducing sugar, avoiding caffeine and cutting out red wine from your diet. Also avoid tyramine, which is found in aged and fermented foods such as old cheeses, smoked fish or cured meats, as it can trigger headaches. Maintain blood-sugar levels by eating regularly and ensure you are getting a few cups of leafy green vegetables most days.
>
> Aim to stay well hydrated by drinking at least 1.5 litres (52 fl oz/6 cups) of water daily; add a squeeze of fresh lemon juice for extra liver support. Herbal teas such as chamomile, lemon balm and lavender can help to soothe a headache and also count toward your daily fluid intake. A bath with Epsom salts (magnesium sulphate) and a little lavender essential oil rubbed gently on your temples can also provide relief from the pain. A naturopath may be able to suggest additional supplements. See your GP if the headaches are unusually strong or frequent, or do not respond to pain relief.

Chamomile, lemon balm or lavender herbal tea

INSOMNIA

Insomnia can be caused by a variety of hormonal problems including disorders of thyroid hormones, testosterone, cortisol and growth hormone. Poor sleep can also be caused by other menstrual symptoms such as pain, bloating and breast tenderness. True premenstrual insomnia, however, seems to be associated with a rapid drop in the relaxing sedative hormone progesterone.[4] This drop occurs just before your period and progesterone levels remain low for the first few days of bleeding. It affects not only sleep onset and sleep maintenance but also sleep quality, which does nothing for mood and energy levels the following day.

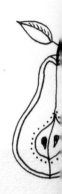

> **TIPS** Ensure good sleep hygiene by creating a consistent bedtime routine to wind down. This means turning off your computer, phones and all devices at least an hour before bedtime. Have a cup of chamomile tea and a warm shower. Dim the lights (try using lamps rather than overhead room lighting) and listen to a short mindfulness meditation before bed. Avoid all caffeine after 10am (including tea).

IRRITABILITY

A few days after ovulation, oestrogen and testosterone levels drop while progesterone rises. This can make some women feel irritable and less focused, while others will feel calmer and more relaxed. The low levels of oestrogen also cause lower levels of serotonin and higher levels of stress hormones such as cortisol, resulting in more irritability, oversensitivity and moodiness. When your period is over, you often feel better due to the increasing levels of oestrogen and testosterone, which can make you feel confident and energised. Women with high oestrogen levels may find they are irritable and anxious around ovulation, so slow down and remember to breathe.

> **TIPS** Deep breathing sounds simplistic, but it can really work. Spend a few minutes three times a day taking 10 slow, deep breaths to push yourself out of fight-or-flight mode and into parasympathetic nervous system dominance. Be prepared: if you know that irritability tends to strike a few days before your period, make a note in your diary to remind yourself it may be happening soon. Having this awareness and forewarning of your emotions can really help.

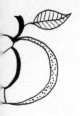

Sugar, caffeine, alcohol, stress and lack of exercise can all impact on irritability in a BIG way, so try to avoid the triggers and stick to a consistent exercise routine. Increase dietary fibre with veggies, nuts and seeds and aim to eat one or two pieces of fruit daily. Ask a naturopath to suggest supplements, and check with your GP if you feel you are not coping with the stress of your emotions.

NAUSEA

Menstrual nausea may be caused by a variety of factors, including pain, hormonal changes, liver function issues and migraines. Normal hormonal changes can result in increased secretion of hydrochloric acid in the stomach, which can cause heartburn, nausea or vomiting. This appears to be worse when eating patterns are irregular. Prostaglandins released by the contracting uterus and associated with pain can also affect the digestive process and contribute to feelings of nausea. Clearance of hormones by the liver is high leading up to menstruation; if liver function is sluggish, it can lead to headaches and nausea.

TIPS Eat regularly and ensure you include protein in all your meals. Snack every three hours and avoid fatty or fried foods. Sip two to three cups of ginger and nettle tea each day to help reduce nausea. If you don't like the taste of ginger tea, you could try ginger tablets for nausea relief. Check with a naturopath. Get plenty of rest but continue gentle exercise such as walking, swimming, yoga and pilates. Some people find that pressing an acupressure point (measure about three finger-widths down your wrist from the base of your hand and press with the opposite thumb) can help. If nausea persists, see a naturopath.

SADNESS

Premenstrual sadness appears to be triggered by low levels of oestrogen and serotonin (our feel-good neurotransmitter). Without these happy hormones, sadness, depression and tears can take over. Extreme depression at this time may be a result of premenstrual dysphoric disorder (PMDD), which is very serious and requires treatment. Of course, most people will experience sadness from time to time, which is perfectly normal and nothing to be concerned about unless it persists.

TIPS Increasing your intake of omega-3 rich foods such as wild-caught fish, eggs, walnuts and chia will go a long way in helping to alleviate the blues. Avoid alcohol. Aim to spend at least 10 minutes in the sun every day. Increase your intake of foods containing tryptophan, the feel-good amino acid: try cottage cheese, spinach, bananas, turkey, seafood and pepitas (pumpkin seeds). Exercise can increase serotonin, which gives you a happy buzz. Be sure you are getting enough calcium: sources include unhulled tahini, parsley, almonds, chia and dried figs. A naturopath may be able to suggest herbal medicine such as St John's wort, passionflower and saffron. If sadness persists, see your GP for a referral for professional guidance.

SALT CRAVINGS

The adrenal glands provide energy, help you cope with stress and are involved in many hormonal processes in the body. When hormonal levels change, the adrenal glands are always working. Adrenal glands require essential minerals to function properly: when we are mineral deficient, we tend to crave salty foods. Common mineral deficiencies are zinc, magnesium, iodine and iron.

TIPS Salt cravings may mean that you are dehydrated or missing out on important minerals, such as zinc, which can be depleted in women taking the oral contraceptive pill[5]. Boost your intake of zinc with pepitas (pumpkin seeds), sesame seeds and nutrient-dense sea vegetables such as nori, kombu and dulse. Satisfy salty cravings with pink Himalayan rock salt or sea salt, sea vegetables or miso soup. Try to avoid processed foods and table salt, which will satisfy cravings but will not restore mineral balance. A naturopath can suggest supplements if they are necessary.

SALT FROM SEA VEGETABLES

Dulse flakes are made from dried seaweed and sold in most health-food stores as a natural flavour enhancer. Dulse has a salty taste and is packed full of fibre, vitamins, trace minerals and antioxidants. Dulse flakes are a rich source of iodine. Try dulse flakes sprinkled over scrambled eggs or popcorn, or add to steamed veggies with a drizzle of olive oil for a tasty side dish.

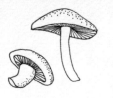

SUGAR CRAVINGS

Cravings for sugar and carbohydrates during your period may be due to a combination of unstable blood-sugar levels, low chromium levels, fatigue and low levels of the happy hormone, serotonin. Sugar is addictive: the more we have, the more we want, which makes having a small treat potentially snowball. Blood-sugar levels can be more variable around menstruation and low blood sugar combined with fatigue often results in sugar cravings as the body tries to improve energy and focus. As mentioned earlier, falling oestrogen levels before menstruation can also result in low serotonin levels. Eating sugar increases serotonin in the brain and releases painkilling beta-endorphins, so it makes us feel good but keeps us wanting more sugar to maintain the feeling.

CROWD OUT SUGAR: FOCUS ON FOODS YOU CAN EAT INSTEAD AND ALWAYS HAVE NUTRITIOUS SNACKS ON HAND.

TIPS Try to avoid all added sugar (check the ingredients on ready-made foods). Stabilise your blood-sugar levels with regular protein snacks every three hours; choose foods that also contain 'good' fats. Suggestions include almond butter spread on apple slices; hummus and celery; cheese and avocado on rice crackers; or natural yoghurt with chia seeds and berries. Increase cardio exercise to release beta-endorphins and eat foods that are high in serotonin such as chicken, kidney beans, bananas, eggs, watermelon and mushrooms. Drinking two cups of cinnamon tea daily may help stabilise blood-sugar levels and further reduce cravings. A naturopath may recommend some other supplements to help reduce sugar cravings.

SPOTTING

Light spotting can occur a few days before menstruation or at the time of ovulation. Some women will experience spotting for longer periods of time and this should always be checked out with your GP, who may recommend an ultrasound to ensure that there are no fibroids or anything else of concern. Premenstrual spotting is usually due to insufficient progesterone levels in the second half of the cycle. Progesterone is responsible for maintaining the uterine lining for pregnancy. When progesterone levels are low, the lining starts to come away before menstruation has begun. This can cause issues for those trying to conceive and is generally annoying for everyone else.

Spotting at ovulation can be caused by oestrogen levels dropping, which can result in a small withdrawal bleed. A single incidence of spotting at ovulation may also occur at the time of follicle rupture, when the egg is released.

TIPS Try to increase your intake of foods containing vitamin B6 such as walnuts, chicken, seafood, bananas, spinach and beans. Progesterone is produced along the same pathway as cortisol so if stress levels are high, progesterone production may be compromised. Manage stress levels by practising mindfulness (see page 98), getting regular exercise and taking time out to breathe deeply. Try to cut down on commitments if you can. See a naturopath for supplements such as vitamin B6 and zinc that may also help support progesterone production.

HEAVY BLEEDING

Heavy bleeding (known as menorrhagia) is experienced by many women but should be investigated when it is a new symptom or is excessive. Some women will bleed so heavily that they leak through super tampons and pads and can experience flooding. Ovarian dysfunction and lack of ovulation may cause heavy bleeding due to insufficient progesterone production. Conditions such as uterine fibroids or polyps should be considered and can be diagnosed via ultrasound. See your GP to rule out serious health issues, especially if this is a new symptom.

Some heavy bleeding may be due to hormonal imbalance (due to high oestrogen, low progesterone, hypothyroidism). When hormones are unbalanced, the lining of the uterus may thicken excessively, which can result in heavy bleeding.

TIPS Assist hormonal balance by reducing your exposure to environmental oestrogens. These are found in plastics, some cleaning products and personal care products. (See pages 88–93 for advice.) Support your liver function by drinking nettle-leaf tea. Eat plenty of organically produced vegetables. Drink three cups of cinnamon tea daily starting from the day before your period is due until the end of your bleed. Ask your GP to check your iron levels.

If your bleeding has been investigated and no underlying condition can be found, a naturopath can recommend a herbal tonic that may help to reduce your heavy blood flow (and make your life easier).

SYMPTOM CHART

DATE:

Day of cycle	1	2	3	4	5	6	7	8	9	10	11	12	13	14	
Menstrual flow															
PMS with mood changes:															
Nervous tension															
Irritability															
Anxiety															
Insomnia															
Crying/sadness															
Depression															
Social withdrawal															
Lack of interest in life															
PMS with food cravings:															
Craving sugar/carbs															
Headaches/migraines															
Irritability if hungry															
Fatigue															
PMS with fluid retention:															
Breast fullness															
Abdominal bloating															
Weight gain															
Swollen hands and feet															
PMS with pain:															
Period pain															
Breast pain															
Aches and pains															
PMS with depletion:															
Tiredness															
Mental fatigue															
Hot flushes															
Headaches/migraines															

Grading of menstruation

0 none
1 slight
2 moderate
3 heavy
4 heavy and clots

Grading of symptoms

0 none
1 mild (only slightly aware, but does not interfere with activities)
2 moderate (aware of symptoms, but does not interfere with activities)
3 severe (continually aware of symptoms, but not disabling)
4 very severe (disabling symptoms, unable to function)

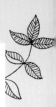

15	16	17	18	19	20	21	22	23	24	25	26	27	28	29	30	31	32	33	34	35	36

COPY
THIS

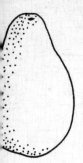

COMMON HORMONAL CONDITIONS

This section gives an explanation of common conditions that can affect hormonal balance and provides diet and lifestyle recommendations to help deal with them. If you think you might be experiencing any of the following conditions, it is advisable to see your GP as well as accessing complementary health care, such as seeing a naturopath.

POLYCYSTIC OVARIAN SYNDROME (PCOS)

PCOS is a hormonal and metabolic condition in which the levels of a woman's sex hormones are out of balance, resulting in a failure to ovulate regularly. This can lead to excessive production of androgens (male hormones, such as testosterone); cysts in the ovaries (visible by ultrasound); and deficiencies of oestrogen and progesterone, which may result in difficulty conceiving. Symptoms may include: irregular or absent menstrual cycles, excess hair growth, acne, poor weight control and fertility issues.

There are several causes of PCOS, many of them overlapping. Insulin resistance — the most common cause of PCOS — is something that can often be corrected with diet and lifestyle changes. Treatment requires time, careful nutrition and may be assisted by naturopathic supplementation. Inflammatory (chronic immune activation) PCOS can also be resolved with proper nutrition and lifestyle changes as described below. Talk to a naturopath before embarking on these changes to make sure you know which ones are right for you.

- The fastest way to regulate your cycle and promote ovulation is by addressing insulin resistance in the ovaries. A low-sugar and low-carbohydrate diet is recommended for women with PCOS. Avoid grains and sugars if your cycle is irregular or missing.

- Focus on protein, 'good' fats and loads of veggies with every meal and for most snacks.

- Minimise your fruit intake: one to two serves per day of low-GI fruits such as berries and cherries.

- Reduce testosterone levels (which may contribute to acne and excess hair growth) with 2–3 cups of spearmint tea daily.

- Aim to exercise four or five times a week to reduce weight (if required) or reduce exercise to two or three times a week if your body weight is very low and exercise frequency or intensity is high. Exercise should include strength and resistance training to build muscle and improve insulin resistance.

- Reduce insulin resistance and stabilise blood-sugar levels by enjoying two to three cups of cinnamon tea daily.

- Increase your intake of magnesium-rich foods such as dark, leafy greens, nuts and seeds.

- Include foods containing chromium, such as broccoli, egg yolks and beans, to reduce sugar cravings.

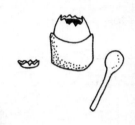

POLYCYSTIC (MULTIFOLLICULAR) OVARIES

The difference between PCOS and polycystic ovaries (PCO) is confusing for many women. PCOS refers to the syndrome described above, while a diagnosis of polycystic ovaries simply means that, in a pelvic ultrasound examination, the ovaries appear to be covered in multiple small follicles. I prefer to call these multifollicular ovaries to limit the confusion. Multifollicular ovaries have an increased number (more than 12) of small follicles that have been arrested during follicle development. They are generally caused by a lack of ovulation and are very commonly seen after prolonged oral contraceptive use, before the woman starts to ovulate and menstruate on her own again. Another cause may be hypothalamic amenorrhoea, which is when the brain stops sending the signals to the pituitary gland to release its hormones and thus overall hormone levels are suppressed and menstruation does not occur.

While most women with PCOS have multifollicular ovaries (due to a lack of regular ovulation), some women with PCOS have ovaries that appear normal. Around 20 per cent of all women having a pelvic ultrasound are found to have multifollicular ovaries and many of these women have regular cycles, ovulate regularly and have normal reproductive function. If the ultrasound was repeated months later, the ovaries would appear normal for many women.

AN ULTRASOUND DIAGNOSIS OF POLYCYSTIC OVARIES SIMPLY MEANS THAT THE OVARIES APPEAR TO BE COVERED IN MULTIPLE SMALL FOLLICLES.

IDENTIFYING AND ADDRESSING
UNDERLYING CAUSES IS MORE
LIKELY TO HELP YOU ACHIEVE
YOUR GOALS AND IMPROVE
YOUR HEALTH OUTCOMES.

Multifollicular ovaries do not usually require treatment unless ovulation is erratic or absent. Causes for this may include use of hormonal contraceptives, hypothyroidism, high levels of the hormone prolactin, breastfeeding, hypothalamic amenorrhoea (when the hypothalamus malfunctions and menstruation stops), eating disorders, excessive exercise, low body weight (or low body fat percentage), acute or chronic stress and some medications. The primary treatment aims depend on the cause of the ovulation dysfunction. Going onto a hormonal contraceptive (such as the Pill) will not make you ovulate or regulate your cycle, just because you seem to be having a period. Identifying and addressing the underlying causes is more likely to help you achieve your goals and improve your health outcomes in the longer term.

If body weight (or body fat percentage) is low and exercise levels are high, start by increasing your intake of 'good' fats including organic eggs, salmon, avocado, nuts and seeds, tahini, coconut oil and olive oil. Reduce exercise to two to three times per week and avoid running and all cardio. Try to think of it as 'movement and circulation' as opposed to 'exercise'. It can be hard, but try giving up boot camp and start gentle walking, yoga or pilates to manage stress and maintain muscle tone.

ENDOMETRIOSIS

Endometriosis is an inflammatory condition with an abnormal immune response, in which the uterine lining grows outside the uterus. This can cause severe pain at any time during the menstrual cycle and should be suspected if the pain is severe, painkillers do not take the pain away or pain interferes with daily activities. Many women also suffer from bowel pain, heavy bleeding and pain with intercourse. See your doctor if you are experiencing these symptoms and try the following dietary changes. The primary aim of these tips is to reduce inflammation and exposure to substances that can increase the level of oestrogen in the body.

- Consume broccoli, cauliflower, asparagus, fennel, kale, spinach and brussels sprouts most days to assist with oestrogen metabolism.

- Avoid heating food in plastic, plastic wrap and plastic water bottles.

- Avoid environmental oestrogen by following the tips in the Lifestyle chapter (see pages 88–93).

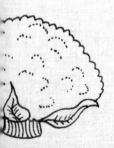

- Avoid dairy, gluten, corn, soy and sugar to reduce inflammation.

- Replace coffee with one to two cups of green tea, which contains antioxidants and may be beneficial.

- Decrease your intake of red meat to around one serve a week (and increase your intake of organic chicken, eggs and fish).

- Try to ensure that most of your food (especially animal products) is organically produced.

- Aim to reduce inflammation by adding turmeric and spices to most meals and consuming LOADS of vegetables every day. At least 40–50 per cent of your daily food intake should be vegetables.

- Add one to two tablespoons of freshly ground linseeds (flaxseeds) to food or drinks daily to add fibre and help eliminate excess oestrogen from your system.

LOW OVARIAN RESERVE

Some women will have a lowered ovarian reserve, measured by the levels of follicle stimulating hormone (FSH), anti-Mullerian hormone (AMH) or an ultrasound follicle count. A lowered reserve means it may be harder to conceive and there may be an increased risk of miscarriage. This will happen naturally as women age, but some women have a low reserve at a younger age. There is still no definitive test for ovarian reserve.

The aim for older mothers or those with low reserve is to protect the quality and quantity of the remaining eggs.

- Avoid alcohol and caffeine.

- Avoid toxic cleaning and body-care products.

- Implement reproductive health lifestyle tips (see the Lifestyle chapter on page 84).

- Increase your intake of antioxidant foods with every meal; try goji berries, chia seeds, blueberries, pepitas (pumpkin seeds), pomegranates, broccoli, pecans, turmeric and fresh herbs.

- Ask your naturopath about supplementing with antioxidant nutrients such as CoQ10, Lipoic Acid and N-Acetylcysteine.

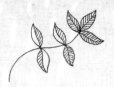

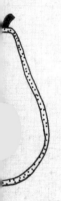

AUTOIMMUNE CONDITIONS

Autoimmune conditions are those in which the body mounts an immune response against its own tissue. These conditions may be specific, such as Hashimoto's thyroiditis, or nonspecific or asymptomatic, such as having elevated levels of antinuclear antibodies (ANAs), antiphospholipid antibodies, or Natural Killer Cells (part of your innate immune system). If your doctor has diagnosed an autoimmune condition, consider making the following dietary changes in addition to your treatment; the aim is to reduce inflammation and support digestive health and the immune system.

- Go gluten free. Gluten antibodies can cross-react with other antibodies, making autoimmune conditions worse.

- Avoid processed foods and added sugar.

- Eat wild-caught fish two or three times a week.

- Aim for 8–10 cups of veggies daily: eat a rainbow of colours and loads of immune-balancing veggies such as shiitake mushrooms.

- Eat organically grown or pasture-fed meats.

- Don't forget to add 'good' fats to every meal, such as avocado, olives, coconut oil, olive oil, tahini, nuts, seeds, pesto.

- Add probiotic-rich foods daily for optimal digestive function (a large part of the immune system is in the gut): fermented veggies, kimchi, kombucha, kefir, miso and yoghurt.

- Try to have a cup of homemade bone broth each day.

- Avoid vegetables that are believed to trigger inflammation such as tomato, capsicum (pepper), white potato, eggplant (aubergine) and chilli.

- Implement regular relaxation and stress management.

- Ensure that you get enough sleep. Try to get eight hours of sleep every night.

- Consider a supplement of good-quality fish oil daily, in consultation with a naturopath.

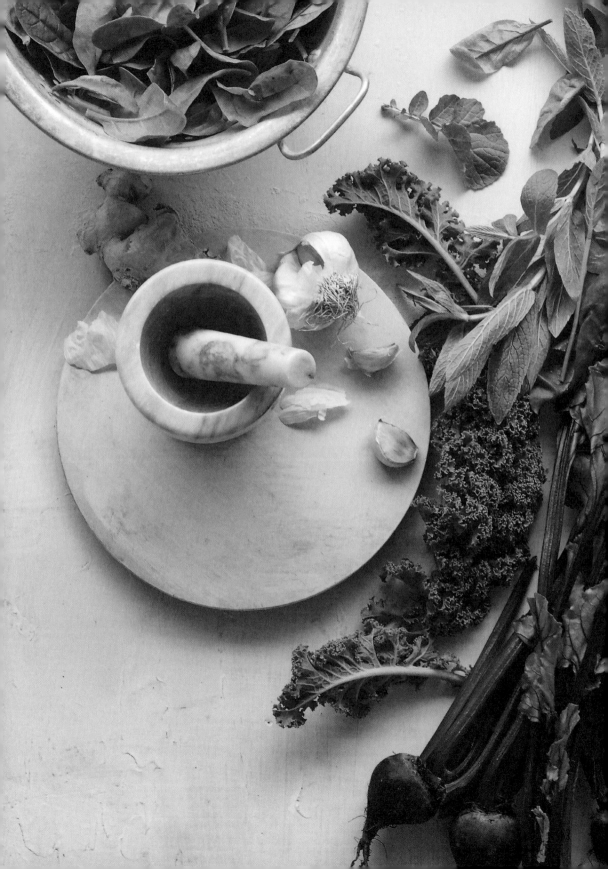

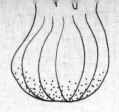

THYROID PROBLEMS

Good thyroid health and function is essential for good hormonal health (and especially for conception and pregnancy maintenance). Your thyroid stimulating hormone (TSH), measured by a blood test, should ideally be lower than 2.5 mIU/L: if it is higher, you may be hypothyroid or subclinically hypothyroid (still within the range of normal, but not optimal for hormonal balance). For a full thyroid assessment, thyroid antibodies should also be checked.

- Gluten can negatively affect thyroid function. Gluten antibodies can cross-react with thyroid antibodies, making autoimmune conditions worse. Try not to load up on gluten-free packaged foods from the supermarket; just focus on eating lots of fresh and unprocessed foods. See the recipes in this book for ideas.

- Avoid soy products, which can depress the thyroid and block the absorption of important nutrients and minerals.

- Cook all broccoli, cauliflower, asparagus, kale, spinach and brussels sprouts to reduce potential negative effects on thyroid function.

- Check your urinary iodine levels (first morning urine) and vitamin D levels — these nutrients are important for making thyroid hormones — and consider asking a naturopath about supplements. Without the right ingredients it's almost impossible for your thyroid to function correctly.

- Eat four or five brazil nuts on most days to increase your intake of selenium, an important mineral for good thyroid health.

GOOD THYROID FUNCTION IS ESSENTIAL FOR GOOD HORMONAL HEALTH (AND ESPECIALLY FOR CONCEPTION AND PREGNANCY).

GENETIC MUTATIONS THAT AFFECT FOLATE ABSORPTION

People with mutations of the gene that produces methylene-tetrahydrofolate reductase (MTHFR) have difficulty metabolising or absorbing folic acid (the synthetic version of folate). This means that folate is not able to easily enter cells and protect DNA, among its many other roles. There are several types of MTHFR mutations and the more severe forms may contribute to a range of negative health effects including miscarriage, mental health problems, fatigue and detoxification pathway issues. Your GP or naturopath can order a genetic test if this condition is suspected.

- Try to avoid synthetic folic acid supplements (in most over-the-counter supplements and conventionally grown wheat products such as bread, cereal, crackers and more). Check product labels.

- Increase your intake of leafy greens for naturally occurring folate.

- Look for a supplement with forms of folate that are already broken down for easy absorption, such as folinic acid and L-methylfolate (or 5-MTHF), and avoid those containing folic acid.

- Try a sauna or an Epsom salts (magnesium sulphate) bath (one cup of Epsom salts per bath) two or three times a week if possible.

- Ensure that you get enough sleep. Try to get eight hours of sleep every night.

- Consult a naturopath about personalised treatment options. People with MTHFR mutations may have adverse reactions to certain supplements.

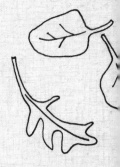

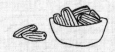

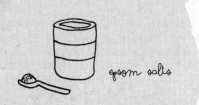

epsom salts

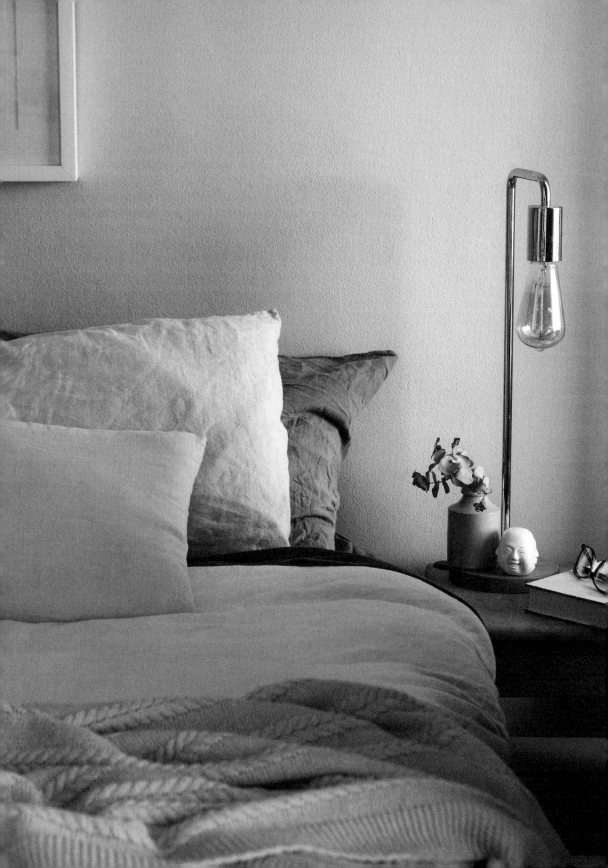

Fertility AND Conception

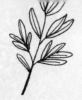

TRYING
to conceive

This special section is for women who are planning conception in the next four months, actively trying to conceive, experiencing fertility problems or have suffered miscarriage.

There is a comprehensive range of pathology tests that you can consider to assess your state of health before trying to conceive. Consult your GP about what tests can be done and ask them to help you understand the results. A naturopath can also order tests, assist you to interpret the results and advise on nutritional supplements or herbal medicines to help you to achieve optimal health and assist with a successful pregnancy and birth. Always inform your GP or specialist if you are using supplements.

If you have been trying unsuccessfully to conceive for six months or more, it's time to see your doctor for further investigations or a referral to a fertility specialist.

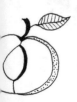

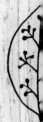

EMOTIONAL ROLLERCOASTER

When you are trying to conceive it can be a time of excitement and anticipation, but it can also be a time of stress and anxiety. The impact of this stress can affect relationships, friendships, finances, sleep quality and more. For those attempting natural conception, sex can begin to feel very clinical and unromantic or men may develop temporary problems with sexual function from the pressure and lack of results. In these situations I usually recommend that couples make an effort to spend some good quality time together and ensure that they are being intimate at times away from the fertile window.

When you have been trying for some time, there can be intense emotional stress: it feels like everyone on social media or all of your friends are magically falling pregnant. Many of your friends or relatives might not even know of your struggles. Even though you are happy for them, it can be really difficult hearing about other people's successes, so please know that you are not alone if you are feeling this way. Sometimes life just isn't fair and that injustice can feel overwhelming. People deal with this in different ways. Be kind to yourself, reach out to your support networks and consider seeing a counsellor or psychologist if you need some extra help.

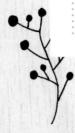

PRE-CONCEPTION

The pre-conception period is widely recognised as being very important to the health of your future baby. Sperm formation can take up to 116 days, and ova (a woman's eggs) take about the same length of time to mature from their primordial state to preovulation. It is recommended that both partners undertake a pre-conception program for a minimum of four months.

Each partner only donates one cell to the potential baby, which means that the health of the DNA in those cells can determine the ultimate health of your baby. It is during the pre-conception time that men have a huge role to play and you can almost think of it as though you are both 'pregnant' during this time.

Pre-conception health care may also help improve fertility in both men and women and assist in increasing the likelihood of a normal, healthy full-term pregnancy; reducing the chance of miscarriage, premature birth and stillbirth; and set you up for a natural unmedicated birth, successful breastfeeding and a happy, healthy baby.

SUBFERTILITY & RECURRENT MISCARRIAGE

Some couples have difficulty with conception or they conceive and then experience miscarriage. It is understood that one in five pregnancies results in miscarriage; in many cases it goes undetected. When couples are told they have 'unexplained infertility', I prefer to use the term 'subfertility', which feels much more positive. Problems can arise from a combination of genetic, environmental, inflammatory and immune components, or there may be specific underlying problems: see our list on page 72.

AFTER TREATING UNDERLYING HEALTH PROBLEMS, MANY COUPLES FIND THEY CAN ACHIEVE THEIR DREAM OF A HEALTHY FULL-TERM PREGNANCY.

By following a pre-conception health care plan, the incidence of miscarriage may be reduced. After investigating and treating underlying health problems, changing diet and lifestyle and implementing appropriate nutritional supplementation, many couples find they can achieve their dream of a healthy full-term pregnancy. There are many tests that may be indicated following miscarriage and it is important to ensure that you are seeing a qualified and experienced practitioner to help you to interpret your results and get the appropriate treatment.

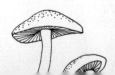

ASSISTED REPRODUCTION

Medical intervention or assisted reproductive technologies (ART) such as in vitro fertilisation (IVF), intrauterine insemination (IUI), intracytoplasmic sperm injection (ICSI) and others may be used for a wide variety of reasons including those listed above. The primary focus during ART cycles is:

- Promoting good egg quality and quantity.

- Providing antioxidants and nutrients for mitochondrial support (giving the embryos adequate energy for growth and cell division).

- Supporting implantation by reducing inflammation and autoimmune problems.

- Ensuring good blood flow, which is essential to embryo survival.

Practical advice for diet and lifestyle:

Increase your intake of antioxidant foods such as turmeric, chia seeds, acai berries, salmon, raw cacao and LOADS of colourful vegetables.

Avoid alcohol and caffeine for three months prior to trying to conceive.

Drink two to three litres (70–105 fl oz/8–12 cups) of filtered water each day.

Try to include a meditation or mindfulness session daily before going to sleep.

Avoid gluten and sugar to reduce inflammation and encourage implantation of the fertilised ovum.

Ensure that you get enough sleep. Try to get eight hours of sleep every night.

Follow the meal plans on page 136 to ensure that each meal contains protein, 'good' fats and plenty of fresh veggies.

Minimise intensive exercise and focus on regular walking and gentle stretching.

Talk to your GP, gynaecologist or fertility specialist and consult a naturopath for further advice.

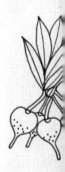

WHY AM I NOT PREGNANT YET?

There are many reasons why conception may be difficult or not immediate.

1. TRYING AT THE WRONG TIME If you know when you are ovulating (use our ovulation chart on page 22), start trying every second day from four days before ovulation to one day after.

2. AUTOIMMUNE CONDITIONS See page 62 for details. Lifestyle and dietary aims are to reduce inflammation, support digestive health and the immune system.

3. STRESS Excessive cortisol production due to long-term or acute stress can affect fertility. This includes people who are always on the go and have very little downtime. Make time to slow down and relax. See our tips on page 81.

4. SPERM QUALITY Sperm quality can be improved by making diet and lifestyle changes. If the male partner is over 35 or you have suffered miscarriages, ask your specialist to test DNA fragmentation of the sperm in addition to semen analysis.

5. THYROID UNDERFUNCTIONING Good thyroid health and function is essential for good hormonal health (especially when it comes to conception and pregnancy maintenance). See page 64 for more information.

6. NUTRIENT DEFICIENCIES Load up on plenty of protein, 'good' fats and vegetables and minimise grains, sugar and processed foods. Follow the Conception Health Diet tips on page 74.

7. LOW BODY WEIGHT Studies have shown that many women with a BMI of 18–19 may still have periods but not be ovulating[6]. Reduce exercise and increase intake of 'good' fats such as avocado, salmon, olive oil and full fat dairy foods.

8. REPRODUCTIVE HEALTH Conditions such as endometriosis, PCOS, fibroids, adhesions and ovulation disorders may be improved with a combination of diet, lifestyle, supplementation and medical treatment (including surgery if required).

9. INSUFFICIENT PROGESTERONE Low progesterone might be an issue if you experience spotting before your period, tender and swollen breasts, PMS or short cycles. Progesterone levels peak a week after ovulation and can be tested with a blood test at this time.

10. MTHFR MUTATIONS There are several types of MTHFR mutations and the more severe forms may contribute to a range of negative health effects including miscarriage and difficulty conceiving. See page 65 for more information.

11. LOW OVARIAN RESERVE This will happen naturally as women age, but some women have low reserves at a younger age. A diet rich in antioxidants, in addition to specific supplementation, can be helpful. You only need one good egg (and one good sperm) but it may take a little longer to find it.

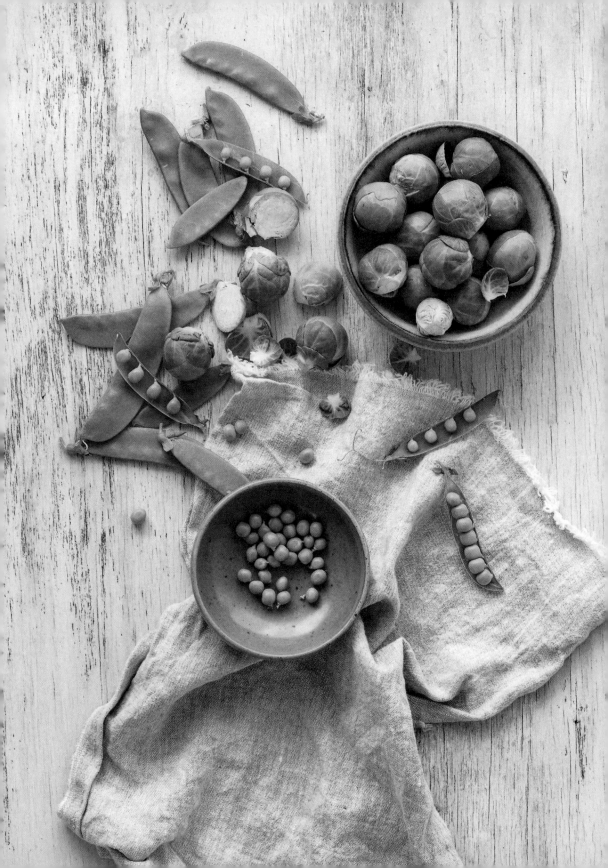

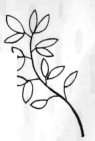

CONCEPTION HEALTH DIET

The conception health diet follows the same principles as outlined in the chapter on Nutrition (see page 100), with just a few small adjustments. The 3–4 months before conception are now considered as important as pregnancy in terms of your nutritional health and the potential effects of environmental toxins and exposure. To begin with, you might like to order an organic fruit and vegetable box each week to help you to eat a variety of fresh, seasonal, organic produce.

For those trying to conceive or planning to conceive in the next three months, it is advisable to avoid large ocean fish such as tuna, shark, swordfish and ling that may be contaminated with heavy metals such as mercury. Avoid tinned tuna and consider replacing it with wild-caught salmon or sardines. Crustaceans and shellfish are often polluted, so try to minimise your intake during this time.

Both partners should avoid alcohol[7] and recreational drugs for at least 3–4 months prior to attempting conception. Avoid smoking and, if you are addicted, take advantage of support, such as nicotine patches, hypnotherapy and psychological help. Cigarette smoke is not only harmful to sperm, egg and embryo development but passive smoking is harmful to the baby after it is born, so it is a good time to make the effort to give up.

Studies have shown that it is important for both partners to reduce or cut out caffeine for at least two months before conception as it is implicated in fertility, pregnancy and baby health problems including miscarriage[8]. Decaffeinated coffee and tea is slightly better, but still not recommended for daily intake during the pre-conception period. Be careful not to replace caffeinated drinks with less nutritious options, such as drinks that contain added sugar. Herbal teas (see page 118) are good substitutes.

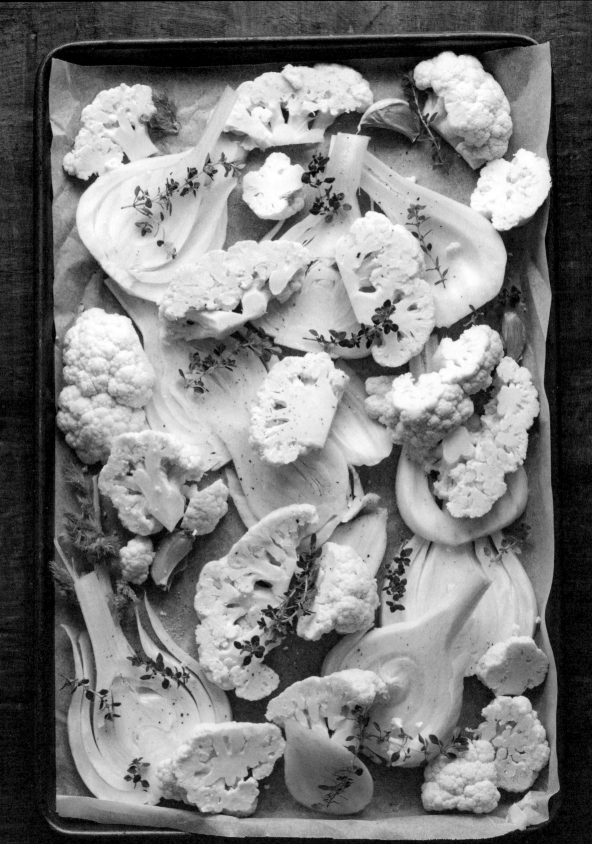

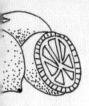

HELPFUL HINTS

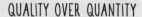

Don't get too caught up in making all these things happen every month, they are just things to be aware of while trying to conceive.

QUALITY OVER QUANTITY

It is important to have regular conception attempts in your fertile window. This is usually around four days before ovulation until one day after. During the days leading up to ovulation and the few days directly after, try to have intercourse every second day. Having intercourse every second day ensures that sperm is fresh.

ELEVATE

Slightly elevate your pelvis directly after intercourse for 15 minutes to help ensure that the ejaculate remains in the cervix for longer. You don't need to have legs up the wall or do crazy-looking bicycle pedalling in the air, just don't jump straight out of bed and clean up. In all honesty, the sperm that is going to get there is probably already at its destination, but you can maximise its chances.

STAY HEALTHY

Increase your intake of vitamin C: it is important to avoid cold and flu tablets and antihistamines while trying to conceive, as they can compromise production of vaginal mucus and seminal fluid.

LUBRICATE SENSIBLY

In cases of cervical damage or dryness, try a sperm-friendly lubricant that adds moisture without harming sperm. A product without added parabens or glycerine is also vagina-friendly.

KEEP IT UP!

It is important to avoid abstinence throughout the rest of the month as regular ejaculation is necessary to keep the sperm fresh and ready for conception. Men should be ejaculating at least every four to five days outside the fertile window.

CONSUME A NUTRIENT-DENSE DIET

See page 136 for some suggested meal plans and use the recipes in this book. Add the top 10 fertility foods (see page 82) to your diet.

EXERCISE REGULARLY

A moderate amount of exercise contributes to optimal health. See page 80 for tips.

IDENTIFY AND TREAT UNDERLYING CONDITIONS

Seek advice from your GP or a reproductive health naturopath and supplement your diet with good-quality nutrients if advised to do so.

KEEP YOUR PELVIC FLOOR TONED

An orgasm, as well as pelvic floor exercises straight after intercourse, can increase chances of conception. Don't worry if you don't orgasm, just squeeze! Pelvic floor exercises will also help during labour and post-delivery, so now there is even more of an incentive to squeeze those muscles!

THINK POSITIVE THOUGHTS

Ensure that you are in a positive frame of mind when you are trying to conceive. Positive visualisations and affirmations are very powerful tools.

DO IT YOUR WAY

Intercourse from behind can also increase chances of conception due to deeper penetration, especially if you have a retroverted uterus. I recommend that couples explore different positions to find out what is most comfortable for them.

TRY TO RELAX

This is possibly the most frustrating thing to say to someone who is trying to conceive, but relaxation techniques such as deep breathing and meditation can be beneficial to conception. Relaxed muscles and increased circulation can help increase the chances of conception and ensure healthy ovulation. If you feel stress building up, that means it's a good time to go for a massage or book a holiday!

REDUCE ALCOHOL AND CAFFEINE INTAKE

See page 74 for more information about the Conception Health Diet.

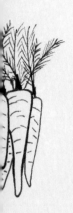

ANTIOXIDANTS

Antioxidants are your cells' protectors, just as paint protects your car from rust or lemon juice prevents a cut apple from turning brown. The process of oxidation causes free radicals to be produced which can damage cells and other structures including proteins, fats and DNA. The body can cope with some free radicals and actually needs them to function effectively; however, an overload has been linked to ageing and disease, in addition to poor sperm and egg health.

Oxidation can be accelerated by many factors, including stress, cigarette smoking, alcohol, over-exercise, medication, sunlight and pollution. Antioxidants can protect the body and help it to repair itself, thus minimising the negative effects of free radicals. The protective effect of antioxidants is essential for good health and keeping eggs healthy for optimal fertility.

The following vitamins and minerals are good sources of antioxidants:

Vitamin C	
berries	mangoes
tomatoes	broccoli
kale	spinach
oranges	capsicum (peppers)
kiwifruit	

Vitamin E	
avocado	olive oil
nuts and seeds	brown rice
dark leafy green vegetables	legumes (beans, lentils, split peas)
sweet potatoes	

Selenium	
brazil nuts	brown rice
chicken	eggs
garlic	onions
seafood	

Betacarotene	
broccoli	kale
spinach	pumpkin (squash)
sweet potatoes	carrots
red and yellow capsicum (peppers)	apricots
rockmelon (cantaloupe)	mangoes

SUPERFOODS

Not all foods are created equal: some are so packed with vitamins, minerals, antioxidants, essential fatty acids and other beneficial substances that they are often called 'superfoods'. The top superfoods listed below should feature regularly in your diet, especially while trying to conceive.

ACAI BERRIES

Acai contains an amazing concentration of antioxidants, amino acids and essential fatty acids. It's considered one of nature's best offerings to combat premature aging, thanks to its high monounsaturated oleic acid content. Oleic acid helps omega-3 fish oils penetrate cell membranes, which helps to reduce inflammation and promote hormone balance. Avoid acai berry preparations that are combined with agave syrup, as this does not promote health.

Acai berry powder is easily sprinkled into smoothies, muesli, yoghurt and muffins.

TURMERIC

Turmeric and other spices such as cinnamon, fennel, chilli, cloves, cumin and ginger are powerful antioxidants; help to reduce inflammation and pain in the body; improve digestion and immunity; and are high in trace nutrients and minerals.

Use it in cooking for a flavour boost or try a Turmeric chai (see page 231).

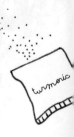

turmeric

GOJI BERRIES

They've been called the most nutritionally dense food on Earth, and they taste something like salty raisins. They are a great source of vitamins B and C, antioxidants and 15 amino acids.

Eat with nuts and seeds or chop up and add to porridge, muesli, salads and baked goods. Goji berry juice is also available.

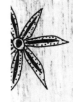

EXERCISE

Exercise in moderation should be your mantra when you start actively trying to conceive. Think of exercise more as movement and circulation rather than sweat and tears. Aim for regular walking and a maximum of two to three exercise sessions a week, which could include yoga, pilates, light weight training or cardio at a moderate intensity. Current recommendations are that adults should be taking a daily average of 10,000 steps per day. If you don't have a wearable fitness device, download a free app to your smartphone and start monitoring your steps. The smartphone won't be as accurate as you probably don't carry it everywhere but it still gives you a good idea of your average step count. If your steps are low, make an effort to take the stairs instead of the lift, park your car a little further away than you need to, get off the bus a stop earlier and go for a short walk in the morning or after dinner in the evening. Combine walking with some gentle bodyweight exercises such as triceps dips, squats, lunges and step-ups for optimal muscle tone and health.

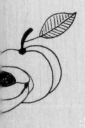

RELAXATION & CONCEPTION

Mindfulness, meditation, visualisation, mantras and setting intentions are all methods of positive psychology to help you to manage stress and maintain your sense of self and happiness throughout the conception and pregnancy process. Start by making time for 10 slow deep breaths on waking and before going to sleep each night. Consider downloading a mindfulness app to your smartphone to help guide you into a relaxed and conception-friendly state of body and mind. For those who like affirmations, write down some positive affirmations and say them aloud in the mirror every day. It can feel a bit silly at first, but it can be a powerful way to keep your mind positive when stress and doubt begin to creep in.

Make time for things that you enjoy and make an effort to slow down the pace of your life. Simple things like eating your breakfast outside, turning your phone off on a Sunday, enjoying a herbal tea in the sunshine or walking with friends in natural surroundings can all help to relax your body and mind. These techniques sound simple and they are: it is making the time and prioritising them that can be difficult, but not impossible.

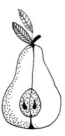

Top 10 fertility foods

1. EGGS – a great source of quality protein. They are also a great way to boost 'good' fats and contain lots of selenium, magnesium, zinc and other vitamins. Eggs also contain choline (a commonly deficient nutrient), which reduces inflammation and supports the process of methylation, which is essential for a full-term pregnancy. You can eat two to three organic eggs every day.

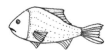

2. SALMON – a great source of protein and good fats, salmon helps to reduce inflammation and promote good hormonal balance. The omega-3s in salmon support baby's brain development and can also reduce the chance of your baby developing allergies. Aim to eat salmon (or mackerel, herring or sardines) at least twice weekly.

3. ASPARAGUS – full of naturally occurring folate and a rich source of glutathione, asparagus is the perfect side dish in your fertility diet. The glutathione in asparagus can help to rid the body of excess oestrogen that may be contributing to period pain, fibroids or endometriosis. It is used in a process called glutathione conjugation in the liver, in which glutathione is added to oestrogen to help its excretion.

4. AVOCADO – a study has shown that intake of monounsaturated fats (the type found in avocados) is related to successful ART pregnancy rates[9]. These fats are believed to improve fertility by lowering inflammation in the body and improving egg and embryo quality. Avocados are high in vitamin E, which is important for egg health in addition to increasing sperm motility and health. Studies have shown vitamin E can be beneficial in improving the uterine lining and can also help with embryo implantation. Avocados are also packed with folate and vitamin B6, which helps to support progesterone levels and implantation. Avocados are a great way to keep you feeling satisfied when you are reducing grains in your diet. Start by eating half an avocado most days.

5. BRAZIL NUTS – a great source of protein and 'good' fats in addition to being a rich source of selenium. Selenium plays an important role in conception (and is often depleted in our overfarmed soils). Selenium is essential for a healthy thyroid and is an important antioxidant. Preliminary studies have shown that selenium may play a part as an antioxidant during egg development and that eggs that resulted in pregnancy contained double the levels of a selenium-carrying protein[10]. I would recommend that all women trying to conceive aim to eat four to five brazil nuts most days.

6. CHIA SEEDS – one of my favourite and most versatile fertility foods, chia seeds are a true superfood containing loads of omega-3s, antioxidants, fibre, iron, magnesium, calcium and potassium. Not only are these tiny seeds packed full of nutrition, they are a great source of complete and highly available protein. The fibre in chia seeds helps to excrete unwanted hormones from the body and keeps the digestive system regular and able to absorb nutrients from the foods you eat. Chia seeds have almost no taste, which means they can be added to almost any meal. Aim for at least a tablespoon of chia seeds most days.

7. PEPITAS (pumpkin seeds) – a super source of the fertility-friendly mineral zinc. In men, zinc can increase sperm count and testosterone levels. In women, zinc is important in helping your body to utilise the reproductive hormones, oestrogen and progesterone. Low zinc can lead to menstrual irregularity and abnormal egg development. When zinc levels are low, protein metabolism is inhibited, which may contribute to lower egg quality. Zinc is commonly depleted in women who have been on the oral contraceptive pill, so if this is you, try to eat a handful of pepitas most days.

8. BEETROOT – fresh beetroot is a great source of resveratrol, the antioxidant that may help in age-related fertility issues. The nitrates in beetroot can be coverted into nitric oxide in the body and may help to improve blood flow, increasing reproductive circulation and supporting egg implantation. Fresh beetroot is also high in fertility-friendly folate, which makes it a great all-round vegetable to include in roasts, salads and smoothies. Note: tinned beetroot is full of salt and sugar and should be avoided.

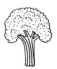

9. BROCCOLI – should be included most days for optimal hormonal health and fertility. Broccoli is a member of the brassica family and contains indole-3-carbinol, which helps the body to get rid of excess oestrogen. Broccoli (in addition to other brassica vegetables such as cauliflower, cabbage, kale and brussels sprouts) can be eaten lightly steamed or baked. It is essential for those with oestrogen-dominant conditions such as endometriosis, fibroids and subfertility. Aim for two cups from this veggie family most days.

10. LEAFY GREENS – including spinach, rocket (arugula), lettuce, watercress, Asian greens, broccoli and fresh herbs, are essential to EVERY fertility diet. Leafy greens are anti-inflammatory and high in naturally occurring folate, the B vitamin that ensures that cells divide, grow and replicate properly. You might be surprised at just how many leafy greens you need to support optimal health and fertility: three cups, most days! This amount is easy to get to if you add them to smoothies, add a handful to your morning eggs, use them in salads and as a base to EVERY dinner. Aim for a wide variety of leafy greens to get the biggest nutrient variety.

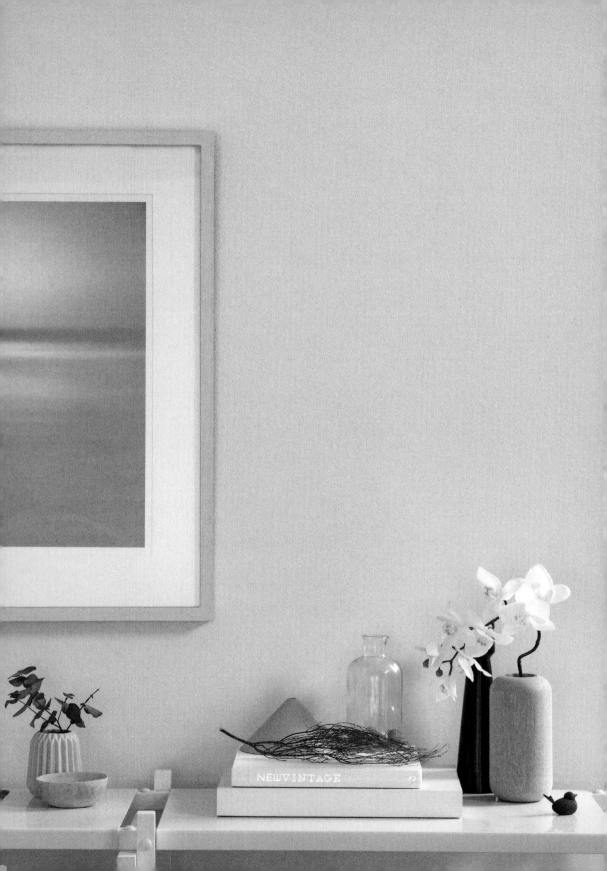

Lifestyle

···

LIFESTYLE TIPS
for hormonal health

Your immediate environment — the food you eat, the products you use, the clothes you wear — are part of a delicate ecosystem that can help or hinder your hormonal balance. The tips in this chapter are designed to help get your hormones into top shape and assist in reducing your overall toxic load, which can increase your wellbeing.

Please remember that this is only a guide: most of us (including me!) can't do all of these things, all of the time. Eliminating chemical cosmetic and cleaning products from your home can take years, so make small changes over time as your budget allows. Organic foods can sometimes be expensive and farmers' markets may not be available in your area, so do your best and remember, it's all about the balance: it's impossible to be perfect!

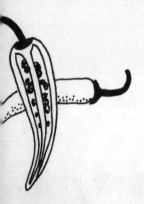

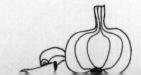

READING PRODUCT LABELS

We are constantly exposed to chemicals. Some chemicals, known as endocrine disrupting chemicals (EDCs) are known to damage hormones. Scientists are increasingly worried that even very low levels of chemical contaminants in the environment may be having significant and long-lasting negative effects on our bodies, particularly on unborn babies. The effects of some chemical exposure during pregnancy have already been shown to affect the health of not only the fetus but also the next generation.

It can be hard to protect yourself from all contaminants in the environment and the air you breathe; however, you can take control of the chemicals you use for personal care, household cleaning and in your garden. We can choose to eat organically grown, unprocessed foods to minimise exposure to pesticides, plastics and other potential dangers. There are some things you can't control, so be proactive and take care of what you can to protect your health and wellbeing and that of your family now and in future generations.

When choosing household and personal products, look for certified organic, nontoxic products. Cosmetics and skincare products can contain unwanted chemicals that may enter the body through skin, hair and nails or as fumes. That even includes some things that smell really good: many perfumes contain synthetic chemical fragrances. Understanding potentially harmful chemicals, where they are hiding and what they might do to us is an in-depth topic you can discuss with a naturopath. Some things to look out for and avoid are listed on the following pages.

LIFESTYLE CHANGES

MAKE AS MUCH OF YOUR DIET ORGANIC AS POSSIBLE. I recommend buying produce from an organic delivery service or checking out your local farmers' market, where the produce sold is usually grown organically or at least is grown locally. This will reduce your exposure to the hormone-disrupting chemicals that are sometimes sprayed on fruits and vegetables. Aim to eat organically produced meat, poultry, dairy foods and butter from animals that are preferably not treated with steroids and antibiotics[11].

ALWAYS WASH FRUITS AND VEGETABLES. It is a good idea to wash and peel your produce to remove any external chemical, organic and wax residues. A fruit and vegetable wash can be purchased from most health-food stores: a simple rinse under cold water often isn't enough to remove fat-soluble residues. You can also try washing your produce in a solution of three parts water to one part apple cider vinegar.

USE FOOD TO BOOST YOUR LIVER FUNCTION AND PROTECT YOUR BODY. Asparagus, spinach, watermelon, pears, pumpkin (squash), potatoes, broccoli, cauliflower and other cruciferous vegetables are rich in glutamine, which can help the liver remove waste and boost your immune system. Increasing your intake of foods that contain allyl sulphide — such as garlic, shallots, onions and chives — also stimulates glutathione production, which further helps to protect the liver and reduce oxidative stress.

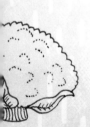

AVOID TINNED FOODS OR FOODS PACKAGED IN PLASTIC. Many plastics and the linings of tins contain bisphenol A (BPA), a chemical that was first identified as a synthetic oestrogen in the 1930s and was even considered for pharmaceutical use at that time. Since that time, BPA has been identified as an endocrine disruptor, and many countries are currently requiring its use to be phased out[12]. Endocrine disruptors may be linked to cancerous tumours, birth defects and developmental disorders[13]. BPA can leach from the lining of a tin into the food it contains. Many plastics also contain BPA and other chemicals, and the softer the plastic, the more likely the chemicals are to leach into food stored in the container. While there is current debate concerning the effects of low-dose exposure to BPA on human health, try to avoid it where possible[14]. Try to have hot drinks in a ceramic mug and avoid using takeaway coffee cups, which have a plastic lid and a plastic lining. Instead of using plastic wrap, you can purchase biofilm from most health-food stores. Use glass cookware for microwave and oven cooking. Practically, most of us will use tinned foods and plastic containers for convenience from time to time, but we can minimise their use and look for alternatives where practical.

INSTALL A WATER FILTER. It is important that water is as fresh and pure as possible, as we drink so much of it! A filter can ensure that there are no unwanted contaminants from ageing household pipes as well as biological contaminants such as parasites[15]. I think it also tastes better.

USE PLANTS FOR FILTERING THE AIR IN YOUR HOME. Some common household plants can help clear the air[16]. The peace lily (*Spathyphillum* spp.) is a low-maintenance indoor plant that helps to reduce mould and clears chemicals such as formaldehyde, benzene and trichloroethylene from the air. The bamboo palm (*Chamaedorea seifrizii*) is also great at improving air quality and helps to put moisture into the air due to its high transpiration rate.

ELIMINATE PESTICIDE, HERBICIDE AND INSECTICIDE use on lawns and gardens. There are many effective organic products available, or you can learn to make your own pest-control formulas. Do an internet search for 'natural pesticides' or ask at your local garden centre. You may also find that planting your garden with species that are native to your country or region makes it easier to look after and requires few, if any, chemical solutions. It's easy to make your own compost as well, rather than relying on mass-produced fertilisers.

AVOID PET PRODUCTS SUCH AS FLEA COLLARS and commercial pet washes, which usually contain toxic substances that may be dangerous to both animals and pet owners. Remember that any product that can kill an insect is also potentially harmful to humans, so avoid using flysprays and other bug killers in the home. There are plenty of more natural options available that are safe for you and your family; try using cedarwood oil products, which can kill fleas and ticks[17].

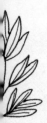

START TO MAKE THE SWITCH TO ORGANIC PERSONAL CARE PRODUCTS.

such as deodorants, shampoos, sunscreens, skin care, body care and baby products. It is easy and cheap to make many personal care products using items from your kitchen cabinet. My all-time favourite eye make-up remover is coconut oil, which is nontoxic, cheap and works brilliantly. Be aware of synthetic fragrances in products, which can be hormone disruptors[18].

AVOID ANTI-BACTERIAL ANYTHING.

The US Food and Drug Administration (FDA) has recently banned the use of several key chemicals in antibacterial hand soap, including triclosan and triclocarban, due to their potentially damaging effects on the immune system. The FDA states that antibacterial washes may not only do more harm than good, but there is also no scientific evidence that they are any better than simple soap and water. I believe that certain ingredients in these products may also contribute to bacterial resistance to antibiotics and have unwanted hormonal effects.

CHECK YOUR SUNSCREEN.

Look for sunscreens with natural ingredients and preservatives and use a physical barrier such as zinc oxide to protect your skin from the sun's harmful rays. It is also a good idea to always wear a hat and stay out of the sun in the middle of the day. Unfortunately, even sunscreen (which protects us from harmful UV radiation) may contain potential endocrine disruptors[19]. Some 'natural' sunscreens also have unnatural preservatives, so be sure to read the ingredient list carefully.

MAKE-UP.

Products you are using on your body and even your lips (where small amounts can be ingested) may contain potentially harmful ingredients. Luckily for us, natural and nontoxic make-up is available, so it is worth doing your research and aligning yourself with brands you can trust. It is important to note that a tiny bit of any of these chemicals is unlikely to cause harm in isolation but when you are using these products on a regular basis, you may end up with levels that are not considered healthy. Check the labels on your make-up and skin-care products and see the table on the opposite page for common ingredients you may want to avoid.

SUBSTANCE	WHY IT'S HARMFUL	COMMONLY FOUND IN
Parabens	Parabens can mimic oestrogen and have been shown to disrupt hormones, in addition to being linked to skin and breast cancers.	Shampoo, conditioner, deodorants, shower gels and facial scrubs.
Phthalates	Two decades of research on phthalates have shown hormonal disruption and potential harm to the unborn baby during pregnancy. Also inked to infertility and reduced levels of sex hormones.	Cosmetics, lotion, nail polish, body wash and hair-care products.
Lead	Neurotoxin linked to hormonal disruption, miscarriage and fertility problems.	Very tiny amounts may be found in lipstick, eyeshadow and foundation.
Quaternium-15	A known skin irritant and allergen that is a special concern for hairdressers and cleaners who may be exposed for long periods of time.	Hair conditioner, hair styling products, shaving products, household cleaning products and some contact lens solutions.
Butylated hydroxyanisole (BHA) and butylated hydroxytoluene (BHT)	These preservatives have been shown to impair blood clotting and promote tumour growth: they are banned in many countries.	Lipstick, eyeliner, blusher, foundation, moisturiser, skin cleanser.
Fragrances derived from petrochemicals	Many products list 'fragrance' or 'perfume' on their label but few disclose exactly which chemicals are used to create the fragrance. Many of them contain phthalates and ingredients that may be hormone disruptors. It's better to be safe than sorry.	Found in nearly every personal-care product: perfume, deodorant, body lotion, soap, shampoo, foundation, sunscreen and also household products such as scented candles, air freshener, detergents and cleaning products.

NAIL POLISH (nail varnish). As consumers make their desire for more natural nail polish products known, many cosmetic companies are offering an increasing range of nontoxic nail polish formulations. These products are marketed as avoiding any or all of the following compounds: dibutyl phthalate (DBP), formaldehyde, toluene, camphor, formaldehyde resin, ethyl tosylamide and xylene. Look for nail polish marketed as 3-free, 5-free or 7-free. While all of these substances can be toxic in large doses, there is as yet no evidence that the amounts you might absorb from nail polish are harmful. Yet sometimes, if you can make the choice to avoid them, it's better to be safe than sorry.

PERFUMES. Many of the chemicals found in perfumes and synthetic fragrances are made from petrochemicals. More than three-quarters of the products that list 'fragrance' as an ingredient contain phthalates, which have been shown to have a negative effect on hormones. Many people notice that perfume gives them headaches or nausea, or that fragrances added to products such as sanitary items, washing powder and toilet paper might cause them irritation. If you are worried about their effects — known and unknown — it is a good idea to avoid synthetic fragrances. It was a sad day when I gave up wearing my favourite perfume, but it did lead me to discover that there are beautiful fragrances made from pure botanical extracts and essential oil blends.

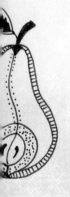

SHAMPOO AND CONDITIONER. Many hair products claim to be 'natural' or 'contain organic ingredients' but may still contain unwanted ingredients. As always, do your research and align yourself with brands that are truly natural and toxin free. The top four ingredients found in shampoo and conditioner and best avoided for optimal hormonal balance include: sulphates, parabens, synthetic fragrances and triclosan (an antibacterial)[20]. Sulphates can be skin irritants and there is some concern about their potential effects over time; they are often found in foaming products such as shampoo, toothpaste and liquid soap.

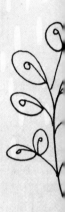

SELF-TANNING SPRAYS AND LOTIONS. Scientific reviews of the active chemical used in many spray tans, dihydroxyacetone (DHA) have shown a potential for DNA damage, and there are concerns over the results of long-term usage[21]. There is an increasing range of good-quality natural self-tanning alternatives on the market. Look for a product that is from a plant or mineral source and does not contain synthetic ingredients. A 'certified organic' logo should guarantee against synthetic ingredients, fragrances and unwanted ingredients.

CHOOSE MILDER HOUSEHOLD CLEANING PRODUCTS. Look for cleaning products that are 100 per cent natural and certified as organic. Alternatively, learn to make your own cleaning products using ingredients such as white vinegar and bicarbonate of soda (baking soda): you will be amazed at how well they work and they might save you money at the same time. The residues of cleaning products can remain in our homes and offices for a long time, leaving us exposed to their effects on a daily basis. I would firstly recommend discarding anything that has a hazard symbol or a warning about the product being a poison, irritant or containing corrosive ingredients. Minimise exposure to products containing synthetic chemicals and look for 'natural' alternatives.

∙∙

THERE ARE BEAUTIFUL FRAGRANCES MADE FROM PURE BOTANICAL EXTRACTS AND ESSENTIAL OIL BLENDS.

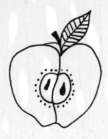

EXERCISE AND HORMONAL BALANCE

Exercise! Sweating eliminates all kinds of chemicals that would otherwise exit the body through your other excretory organs (such as the bladder and bowel). Exercise also calms the mind and gives a good happy hormone buzz, which can only be beneficial for your health, right?

Exercise will generally have a positive effect on hormonal balance. Indeed, exercise and physical activity have been shown to decrease circulating sex hormones independent of any weight loss, making physical activity a must for most, in particular those with oestrogen or testosterone excess. Exercise can also help to reduce stress and decrease the release of cortisol, which can be a contributing factor to progesterone deficiency. In terms of fertility, research has shown that regular, moderate exercise positively influences fertility and IVF outcomes[22]. One hour of moderate exercise three times weekly can improve rate of implantation and reduce risk of miscarriage.

Being overweight or obese can disrupt hormonal balance and impair fertility. Increased body weight can cause irregular ovulation and irregular menstrual cycles. Fat cells, known as adipose tissue, contain an enzyme called aromatase that can increase levels of oestrogen, possibly contributing to hormonal imbalance.

As with anything, moderation is the key. There can also be negative effects of high-intensity exercise on hormonal balance and fertility. Numerous studies have shown that frequent, high-intensity workouts, such as running and frequent bootcamp-style workouts, can reduce oestrogen, disrupt ovulation and cause regular periods to cease. If you are very athletic you may have lower levels of body fat and reduced oestrogen levels. In my clinic, I often need to encourage women to exercise less to improve their fertility or regulate their menstrual cycles. This can be quite difficult as the love of and addiction to exercise is often very strong and it can be difficult to understand how something so 'healthy' can be causing problems.

For optimal hormonal balance, aim to exercise four to five times a week to reduce weight if required, or do high-intensity exercise a maximum of two or three times a week if your body weight is very low. Mixing high-intensity sessions with yoga, pilates, walking and rest days is a great way to keep your fitness levels up while you regain hormonal balance.

It can be really confusing to know what type of exercise is best for you. Exercise can really heal or harm your cycle so it's best to get professional advice if you are unsure. If you are suspect you have a hormonal imbalance or are currently trying to conceive, try to take a very moderate approach to exercise. Focus more on movement and circulation and less on endurance and high intensity. If you are not exercising, it's time to begin, slowly and gently.

Exercise is great for stress relief, but a big workout can increase your cortisol levels and decrease progesterone, which is essential for a regular menstrual cycle, good mood and early pregnancy maintenance. Aim to exercise for just 30 minutes at a time and try interval training, which can reduce exercise intensity to keep your cortisol levels low[23].

For those who are exercising frequently or at a high intensity, and are not experiencing any issues with hormones, immunity or energy and are not trying to conceive, feel free to keep doing what you love. Listen to your body and remember that there is never a one-size-fits-all approach.

Women with a sedentary lifestyle often have a higher percentage of body fat and a lower percentage of lean muscle, which is associated with oestrogen excess and conditions such as polycystic ovarian syndrome (PCOS). Moderate exercise is also essential for promoting blood flow to the reproductive organs, which can assist fertility and reduce symptoms of menstrual pain and inflammation. If you are currently not exercising, aim to increase your daily step count (which you can monitor on your smartphone or tracking device) by going for a short walk most days and commit to one yoga class, or similar, per week. As this becomes part of your normal routine, increase the steps, try some light interval jogging and aim for two yoga classes (or similar) each week.

MODERATE EXERCISE IS ESSENTIAL FOR PROMOTING BLOOD FLOW TO THE REPRODUCTIVE ORGANS, WHICH CAN ASSIST FERTILITY AND REDUCE SYMPTOMS OF MENSTRUAL PAIN AND INFLAMMATION.

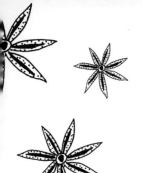

STRESS

Stress can impact nearly every area of health and wellness, including our hormones. The sympathetic nervous system is designed for fight-or-flight and focuses on immediate survival, which does not include reproduction. When the sympathetic nervous system is activated in a stressful situation, production of oestrogen and progesterone decreases and ovarian function may be suppressed. When you have chronic stress, levels of stress hormones remain high.

TIPS Balance chronic stress and an overactive sympathetic nervous system by focusing on stress reduction. Learn to say no and stop overcommitting yourself; laugh daily; try a short mindfulness session (use an app on your smartphone) before bed each night; make time for regular walking; minimise caffeine, sugar and alcohol; and ensure you are eating a nutrient-dense diet. Licorice tea is great for supporting adrenal gland health so try to drink two cups most days. Consider an appointment with a naturopath for nutritional and herbal supplements that may help you manage stress.

THE SYMPATHETIC NERVOUS SYSTEM IS DESIGNED FOR FIGHT-OR-FLIGHT AND FOCUSES ON IMMEDIATE SURVIVAL. WHICH DOES NOT INCLUDE REPRODUCTION.

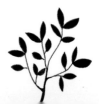

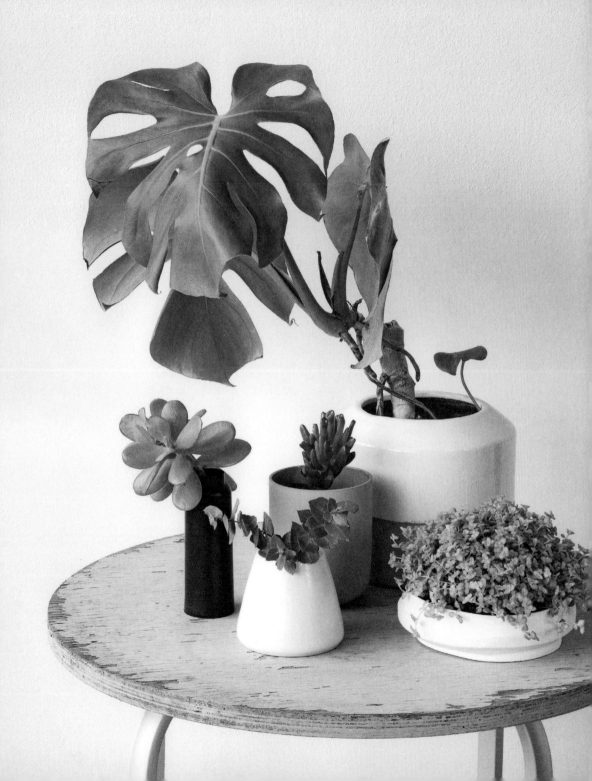

MEDITATION
AND *mindfulness*

Making time to slow down and be mindful is an essential part of a healthy lifestyle in the modern world. Meditation and mindfulness can help to reduce stress and the negative impact of cortisol on hormonal balance; they also promote healthy moods, good immunity and restful sleep. The great thing about incorporating mindfulness and meditation into your regular routine is that the practice doesn't have to take long, it can be done anywhere, it costs nothing and you can't get it wrong. Simply trying to be mindful and meditative slows down the body, increases parasympathetic nervous system activity, decreases excessive cortisol and reduces inflammation.

Studies have shown that mindfulness is linked to positive changes in the brain and the body's production of hormones. In addition to its physical effects, mindfulness may also reduce the emotional experience of pain, making it essential for those with chronic pain conditions such as endometriosis. There is a theory that high cortisol levels can decrease the production of progesterone and result in a relative progesterone deficiency or relative oestrogen excess. This may exacerbate negative menstrual symptoms and, in cases of severe or chronic stress, even delay ovulation.

Any type of meditation or mindfulness can help to reduce anxiety and reduce cortisol levels. Even taking a few slow deep breaths activates the vagus nerve to send a message within your nervous system to lower blood pressure, slow the heart rate and decrease cortisol. Try it right now: close your eyes and take 10 slow, deep breaths and feel the difference within yourself. I recommend that my clients get into the habit of destressing by listening to a meditation or mindfulness app on their smartphone for 10 minutes before bed each night.

THE IMPORTANCE OF SLEEP AND REST

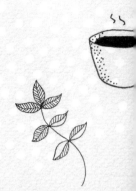

Adequate sleep is essential for good health and happy hormones. Unfortunately, we often sacrifice sleep time for work, household chores and leisure time.

Most experts agree that women need an average of seven to nine hours of sleep each night for optimal health. When the body does not spend enough time in REM sleep (a stage of sleep characterised by Rapid Eye Movement), many believe it can have a negative effect on general health, resulting in hormonal disruption, irregular menstrual cycles and delayed ovulation. Insufficient sleep can also affect weight loss or gain. When we have had enough to eat, a hormone called leptin signals to the brain that we are satisifed and suppresses our appetite. Regular sleep is needed to produce leptin and sleep loss is associated with an increase in appetite and weight gain[24]. Leptin levels can also affect ovulation, so disrupted leptin release due to lack of sleep can lead to irregular menstrual cycles.

The answer? Prioritise your sleep time. Try to create a sleep routine in which you go to bed at the same time each night and wake at the same time each morning.

SOUND SLEEP TIPS

Aim to exercise early in the day

Make your bedroom as dark as possible; dim bright lights in the evening

Reduce clutter and electronic devices from beside your bed

Avoid television, computers and smartphones for at least half an hour before bed

Drink a cup of chamomile or valerian tea just before bed

When you lie down to sleep, take 10 deep, slow breaths with your eyes closed (or use a mindfulness app on your smartphone)

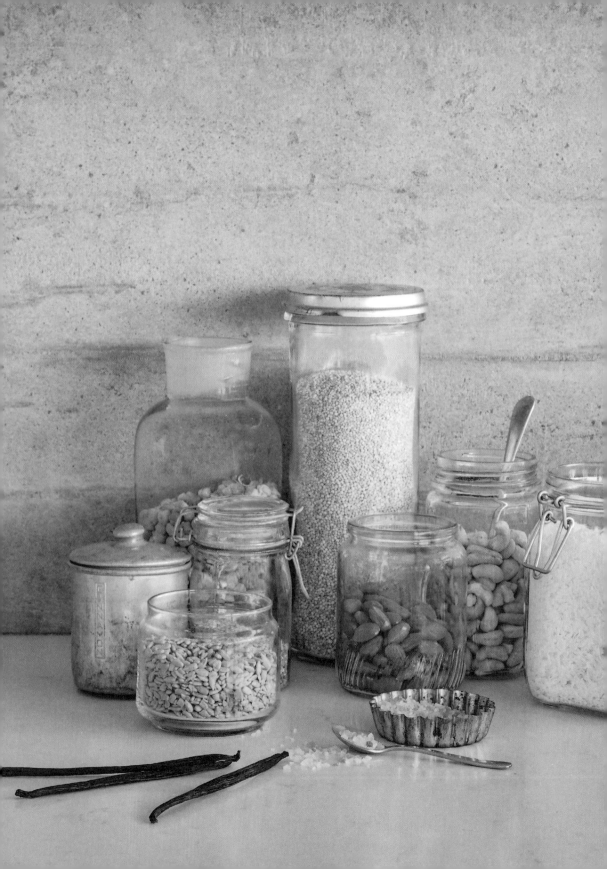

Nutrition

······································

NUTRITION FOR
hormonal balance

Good food choices help to nourish the body and poor food choices can be harmful. Not only do low-nutrient foods take the place of nutrient-dense foods, they can also cause inflammation, immune reactions and tissue damage. The occasional treat is fine, but make sure that nutrient-poor foods are not a regular part of your daily diet. The 80–20 rule, whereby 80 per cent of your diet is based on nutritious wholefoods and 20 per cent is reserved for treats, is usually a good rule to follow for general health. You could even try to follow a 90–10 plan if you are working on improving a specific condition.

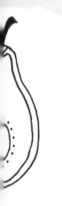

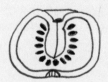

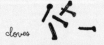

cloves

Crowd out less nutritious food choices by concentrating on the foods that are good for you. If you focus only on the foods you shouldn't eat, you will feel deprived and start craving them even more. Instead, focus on the foods you can eat and enjoy. Eating well is all about organisation and preparation. Make a weekly meal plan (including snacks) and shop and prepare in advance. When you are eating regularly and have tasty meals and snacks on hand, your blood-sugar levels and energy will remain more stable and you are less likely to have cravings. Change your attitude to food: try to see the days when you don't make great food choices as 'less-organised days' rather than 'bad days'.

If long-term health and wellness is a priority for you then you need to change your focus and food choices. You don't have to aim for a perfect diet, but better food choices will become easier with time and practice. Start making time today.

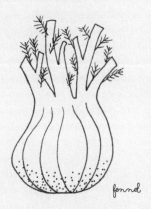

fennel

WHOLEFOODS ARE FOODS THAT ARE AS CLOSE TO THEIR NATURAL STATE AS POSSIBLE. THEY HAVE UNDERGONE LITTLE PROCESSING OR REFINING AND CONTAIN NO ADDITIVES OR ARTIFICIAL INGREDIENTS.

DIGESTIVE HEALTH

Good digestive health is something that many of us take for granted. For those who are not so lucky, it can often be very difficult to isolate foods that make us feel gassy, bloated and uncomfortable. When we feel this way, it is a sign that our digestive system has become inflamed due to the incomplete breakdown of food in the digestive tract. A naturopath can suggest supplements that may be effective in reducing inflammation and healing the digestive system.

CROWD OUT LESS NUTRITIOUS FOOD CHOICES BY CONCENTRATING MORE ON THE FOODS THAT ARE GOOD FOR YOU.

When digestion isn't feeling great (and also during times of convalescence or illness), our digestive systems function better on warm foods: foods that have been cooked and partly broken down, such as soups, stews, casseroles, stewed or soft fruits, nut pastes, porridges and steamed vegetables. To these foods you can add herbs and spices such as ginger, cloves, basil, rosemary, fennel, dill, anise, caraway, cardamom, cumin, parsley and mustard greens. These contain antioxidants and also aid digestion.

Herbal teas are great, both between and after meals. Try fennel, licorice, nettle, peppermint, ginger and chamomile teas to aid digestion.

When your digestion is not at its best, try to minimise salads (especially uncooked leaves), hard and raw fruits (particularly apples), whole nuts and undercooked vegetables, although these things are all are part of a nutritious diet when digestive function is optimal.

In terms of hormones, poor digestive health can reduce the excretion of oestrogen from the body[25]. This can cause symptoms such as mood swings, period pain and heavy bleeding. When the gut is healthy and the diet contains adequate amounts of fibre, oestrogen binds to fibre in the digestive system and is able to be easily excreted. Make sure you include leafy green vegetables, broccoli, chia seeds and linseeds (flaxseeds) in your diet to ensure plenty of fibre.

Foods that stimulate bile production will also help to increase the excretion of cholesterol-based hormones such as oestrogen. Artichokes, rocket (arugula) and other bitter green leaves, sauerkraut, kimchi and other fermented veggies are great for stimulating bile production. Drink one or two teaspoons of apple cider vinegar diluted with 150 ml (5 fl oz) of water before meals.

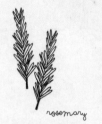

rosemary

WHAT SHOULD I BE EATING?

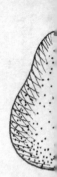

Try to eat a nutritious wholefood diet that includes proteins, 'good' fats and something fresh (fruits and vegetables). Each meal should ideally comprise these three elements, as should most snacks.

Eating in this way means that you don't need to be obsessive or count calories, but allow your body to regulate its own need for food. When we fill up with nutritious foods, we are less likely to overeat; however, when we eat foods that are void of nutrition, our body feels 'hungry' and keeps asking for food. Think of a time when you ate four slices of toast with jam (jelly) and still felt unsatisfied. If you had eaten one piece of toast loaded with avocado, spinach, parsley and egg instead, would you still have been hungry?

The food group not included in the 'protein, "good" fats and something fresh' advice is carbohydrates, or grain-based foods. These foods tend to fill you up, but don't contribute much nutritionally. If you choose to include grains in your diet, make sure they are the accompaniment to the meal, not the basis of it.

The positive psychology of focusing on foods you should include is much better than thinking about the foods you should avoid. Most people are aware that sugar, processed foods, soft drinks, biscuits (cookies), fast food, excess alcohol and caffeine are not very nutritious. These foods are often eaten for convenience or when blood-sugar levels drop and it is hard to make a rational choice. When you plan and prepare what you are going to eat in advance, then blood-sugar levels, mood and energy are more stable, making sugar cravings or junk-food binges less likely.

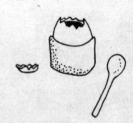

· ·

EVERY MEAL SHOULD IDEALLY COMPRISE PROTEINS, 'GOOD' FATS AND FRESH FRUIT OR VEGETABLES.

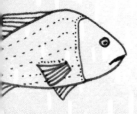

KEY FOODS TO INCLUDE

PROTEIN

Protein is found in animal products (beef, lamb, chicken, turkey, fish, eggs and dairy products) and plant foods (nuts, seeds and legumes). The protein found in plant foods is not quite as easily used by the body as protein from animal sources so, if you follow a mostly plant-based diet, try to include a few types of vegetarian proteins in each meal. It's a good idea to include some form of protein in every meal and most snacks. The need for protein increases during the reproductive years and it is essential for energy and a healthy mood.

Please note that the information about each type of protein below is for general information and to give you food for thought. It's not designed to be a set of strict rules that you must follow, just some general guidelines. I truly believe that a balance of optimal options with some conventional and easy-to-source foods is absolutely fine for most women. A focus on fresh wholefoods is the most important take-home message, and any of the foods listed below are better than eating nutrient-poor foods such as sugary cereals or plain pasta. Focus on the positive.

FISH Aim to include fish in your diet two to three times per week. Locally caught deep-sea fish, such as snapper, trevally, flathead, leatherjacket, whiting, rainbow trout, cod, perch, sea bass, sardines and whitebait, are ideal. If you can find sustainable wild-caught fish it's the better option. Do some research to find a good fish shop in your area and speak to the fishmonger about the fish sources. Many people don't eat fish regularly, as they find it difficult to source fresh fish. Aim to buy fresh fish once a week and freeze a couple of portions for later in the week. The frozen portions work well in curries and fish cakes.

Salmon is a great source of omega-3 and is really easy to cook; however, most commercially available fresh salmon has been farmed. In some circumstances, farmed salmon has been revealed to contain questionable levels of contaminants such as antibiotics, synthetic pigments to improve the colour of the fish and chemicals such as copper, which is used to keep the nets free of algae. The farming process does, on the other hand, minimise the risk of the mercury

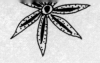

contamination that often affects larger ocean fish. It is possible to buy wild-caught Alaskan salmon which, in Australia, can often be found in the freezer section of health-food stores. It is an expensive option and you may also find organically farmed salmon in the same place, at a cheaper price. I recommend eating commercially farmed salmon no more than once a week. Most tinned salmon is wild-caught and can also be consumed weekly. Salmon, being lower down the food chain and a smaller fish, is less likely to be contaminated with heavy metals than tuna, for example, which is a larger fish.

I generally advise people to avoid large fish such as tuna, shark, swordfish and ling, which may be contaminated with heavy metals such as mercury. That doesn't mean you can't have them every so often at a restaurant. Tinned tuna should be eaten no more than once a week and ideally rotated or replaced with tinned salmon.

POULTRY Aim to include chicken in your diet a maximum of two to three times a week. Conventional chickens are raised intensively to be ready for consumption in 35–55 days, whereas organic chickens are allowed to mature for 65–80 days.

Free-range does not necessarily equate to organic. Free-range chickens are somewhat better for you, as they do roam free; however, they may still be fed antibiotics and other additives in their food. Organically farmed chickens have not been in contact with antibiotics, herbicides or fertiliser residues, which may be hormone disruptors. Aim for organic where possible and be aware that most of the chicken you consume from takeaway sources will have been conventionally raised. This is another reason to make an extra portion of dinner, to save you buying lunch at work the following day.

EGGS Eggs are an excellent source of protein, 'good' fats, vitamins and antioxidants. They help to keep you feeling satisfied and are a quick and easy way to add good-quality protein to your daily diet. Luckily, the myth that eggs increase cholesterol has been scientifically debunked, which means that you can enjoy two to three whole eggs daily. As with chicken, there is a wide price variation between conventional, free-range and organic eggs. In the interests of health and animal welfare, I avoid conventionally raised eggs and opt for organic where possible. 'Pastured' or free-range eggs are nutritionally superior and boast higher levels of omega-3 fats, more vitamins A and E, more betacarotene and less saturated fats. If you can find a local supplier of farm-fresh certified-organic eggs, you are onto a winner.

> A FOCUS ON FRESH WHOLEFOODS IS THE MOST IMPORTANT TAKE-HOME MESSAGE.

Personally, chicken and eggs are the two foods that I never eat if they are not organic and I would urge you to do the same. If the price is an issue, eat organic eggs less often and rotate them with more cost-efficient forms of protein, such as legumes, tahini, nuts and seeds.

DAIRY FOODS Dairy intake is thought to create an excess of oestrogen in the body, which comes from the high oestrogen levels of the dairy cow itself. While the practice is banned in many countries, including Australia, New Zealand, Canada and parts of the EU, in the US, for example, a small proportion of dairy cows may be given synthetic hormones to increase milk production[26]. Some people also experience negative digestive symptoms after consuming dairy products, and it is also linked to acne, blood-sugar irregularities, allergies and hormonal imbalance.

A major source of animal-derived oestrogens in the human diet is milk and dairy products, making these products less desirable for those trying to minimise their oestrogen exposure[27]. Some studies have linked dairy foods to impaired fertility and lack of ovulation in some women, as well as polycystic ovarian syndrome (PCOS)[28].

For those who tolerate dairy foods, it can be part of a balanced and healthy diet. Organically produced dairy products from jersey cows, which produce A2 protein, are preferable if you can get them. A2 protein is genetically different to A1 and A2 protein is considered to be less inflammatory and easier to digest than A1 protein[29].

WHY DO PEOPLE AVOID DAIRY?

Many people are intolerant of dairy products and many women find that avoiding these foods reduces menstrual symptoms such as period pain, heavy periods, acne, PMS and endometriosis.

While some women will have no problems with a moderate level of good-quality dairy consumption, it may be worth doing a three-month dairy-free trial. After the three months are up, some people will experience great results and others may not notice a difference. Listen to your body: this journey is about working out what is right for you, not simply avoiding foods because research or your favourite celebrity says so.

Rotate cow's milk dairy products with sheep's and goat's milk products; these also naturally contain A2 protein and are often better tolerated by the digestive system. Try to use full-cream (full-fat) products, as they are less processed and contain important fat-soluble nutrients such as vitamins A, D, E and K, which are essential for hormone balance, better immunity and the transport of calcium into bone. Low-fat dairy products are a little like white bread: super-refined and missing all the good stuff. If you don't enjoy the taste of full-cream milk, simply dilute it with water. Interestingly, numerous studies have shown that people consuming full-fat dairy products have better weight-loss results and health benefits than those consuming low-fat dairy products[30].

Other dairy food choices include natural yoghurt, kefir, goat's feta, parmesan cheese and butter from grass-fed cows. Note that most cows in Australia and New Zealand are grass fed, but may also be fed supplementary grains. In the USA, most dairy cows are grain fed.

RED MEAT Red meat (beef, lamb, pork and game meats) is a rich source of protein, iron and zinc that can be enjoyed by most people two to three times a week. Look for pasture-raised meats that are also organically farmed. (When animals are grass-fed and roaming around, they produce a higher amount of the 'good' omega-3 fats and less of the inflammatory fats produced by grain-fed animals.)

Slow-cooking and roasting of red meat can make it easier to digest and minimises the potentially harmful carcinogenic side effects of grilling or barbecuing meat. Slow-cooked meat allows you to use traditionally cheaper cuts from a higher-quality source. It seems that excess meat consumption has been linked to endometriosis and should be minimised to once weekly for those with the condition.

Many people who eat a lot of red meat also have a lower vegetable and dietary fibre intake, which may account for some of the negative impact; there is evidence that this unbalanced diet raises oestrogen levels and does not encourage the growth of healthy gut bacteria. Try reducing your portion of red meat at each meal and increasing the amount of fibrous vegetables that you eat alongside it.

It's also a good idea to minimise processed meats, such as salami and ham, unless you are sure of their source and ingredients.

THE POSITIVE PSYCHOLOGY OF FOCUSING ON FOODS YOU SHOULD INCLUDE IS MUCH BETTER THAN THINKING ABOUT THE FOODS YOU SHOULD AVOID.

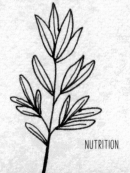

LEGUMES AND PULSES Legumes and pulses are a good source of plant protein and fibre and can add inexpensive vegetarian protein to your diet. Legumes include split peas, lentils, chickpeas (garbanzo beans), kidney beans, cannellini beans, borlotti beans, lima beans and butter beans. Legumes add extra bulk and nourishment to salads, soups and casseroles.

Legumes contain FODMAPs (fermentable oligosaccharides, disaccharides, monosaccharides and polyols). These are types of carbohydrate that are poorly absorbed by some people, resulting in bloating, gas and digestive upset. Legumes also contain phytic acid, which can bind to minerals in food such as iron and zinc and reduce their absorption. Phytic acid can also inhibit enzymes used by the body to break down proteins and starch. Luckily, phytic acid can be partially neutralised by soaking legumes (except red lentils, which don't need soaking) at room temperature overnight. If legumes are prepared correctly and you enjoy and tolerate them, eat them several times a week.

NUTS AND SEEDS Nuts and seeds are a great way to boost your intake of protein and good fats; however, you can have too much of a good thing: around one third of a cup of mixed nuts and seeds is enough each day. Nuts and seeds are so versatile: they can be used in stir-fries, smoothies and salads or as a snack. Rotate the types you buy for maximum nutrient variation and try to always add seeds to your nut mixes for an extra boost. Nut butters are easily found in the health-food aisle of your supermarket and are seriously delicious. My all-time favourite snack is sliced apple dipped in almond butter: it's the perfect combination of protein, 'good' fats and something fresh.

Like legumes, nuts and seeds contain phytic acid (see above), so if you are consuming them regularly it is a good idea to soak them overnight in salty water and rinse thoroughly in the morning. The soaked nuts are then ideally dried in the sun, a dehydrator or in the oven on a very low temperature. This process is also known as 'activating'. Personally, I often skip the drying part, but then you must be careful to only soak what you will consume the following day, to avoid mould from developing.

Always choose raw, unsalted and fresh nuts and seeds. They should not taste bitter or rancid and are best stored in the fridge to keep them fresh. Try a mixture of chia seeds, almonds, brazil nuts, cashews, pecans, walnuts, macadamia nuts, sunflower seeds, pepitas (pumpkin seeds) and sesame seeds: there are so many to choose from. Varieties with particular hormonal benefits include brazil nuts, hazelnuts, walnuts, chia seeds and pepitas (pumpkin seeds).

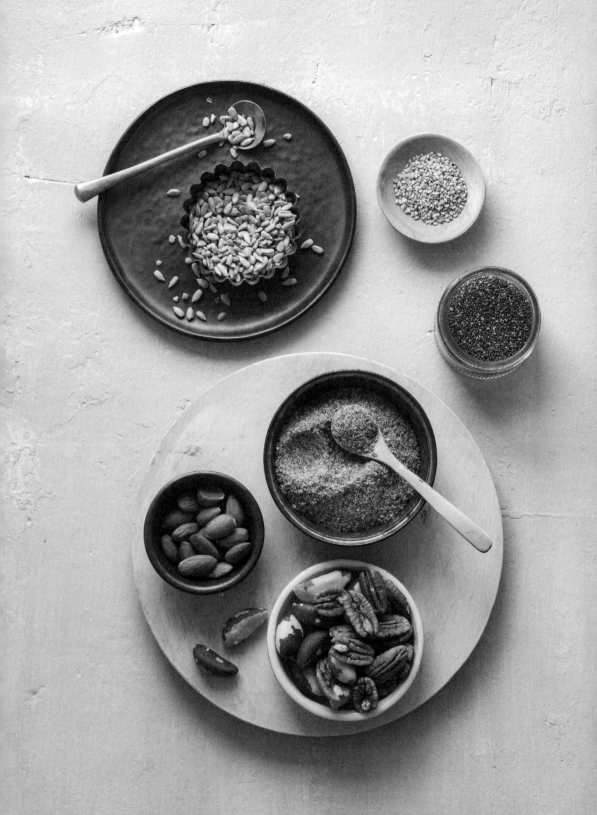

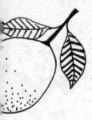

FATS

Many hormones are fat-soluble, so ensure you are including a source of 'good' fats with most meals. 'Good' fats such as those listed below are also essential for satiety (feeling satisfied after a meal) and are particularly important for people following a low-grain diet. Foods containing 'good' fats include olive oil, coconut oil, ghee, avocado, pesto, ricotta cheese, hummus, tahini, nuts, seeds and nut spreads.

Use cold-pressed oils, such as extra virgin olive oil, avocado or macadamia oils, as dressing on salads. When they are not heated, these oils are high in beneficial fatty acids which are essential for hormonal balance. Cold-pressed oils can also be drizzled over veggies after cooking as an easy way to make steamed veggies more appealing. These oils should be kept in a cool, dark place and not kept beyond their use by date. Add lemon, garlic and herbs to your favourite oil to make a yummy salad dressing.

Good-quality organic butter from grass-fed cows is a good source of fat-soluble vitamins including vitamins A and D. Check the label to ensure that no vegetable oils are added to the butter for softening.

The best oils for cooking on the stovetop include coconut oil, butter or ghee. Olive oil can be used for baking in the oven.

Avoid 'bad' fats, which include those found in seed oils, vegetable oils, margarine and trans fats. These are often found in deep-fried food, bakery goods, cinema popcorn and many packaged or processed foods. Synthetic fats, which are added to low-fat products to enhance the texture, are also 'bad'[31]. 'Bad' fats cause inflammation and may contribute to the development of chronic diseases[32].

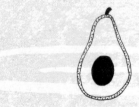

WILL FAT MAKE ME FAT?

Low-fat foods are not wholefoods. Removing fats removes the fat-soluble vitamins A, D, E and K. These vitamins are essential to help absorb calcium and support immunity. Eaten in moderation, 'good' fats should not cause weight gain, but fats are energy-dense, so if you are not burning off that energy you may find that your weight increases.

'Bad' fats are often responsible for unwanted weight gain and inflammation. Many types of 'bad' fats are hidden in foods that do not appear fatty. Crackers, toasted muesli, cake mix and popcorn are examples of foods that appear dry but contain harmful vegetable oils and trans fats, which can disrupt hormonal balance and contribute to weight gain.

SOMETHING FRESH

VEGETABLES You can't get enough fresh vegetables! Aim to eat an abundance of vegetables every day and a wide variety. Ideally we should consume seven different types of vegetables daily, of all colours, equal to about four to five cups of fresh, uncooked veggies. Vegetables can be enjoyed both raw and cooked. Be careful of relying too heavily on salads as your source of fresh food as you may find you are missing out on hormone-balancing vegetables such as broccoli, cauliflower, asparagus, cabbage, fennel, spinach, brussels sprouts and kale, which should be lightly cooked and eaten regularly. When cooking veggies, try a variety of methods: steamed, stir-fried, baked or blanched. Avoid overcooking vegetables as this reduces vitamin levels.

The easiest way to boost your daily vegetable intake is to double the quantity when preparing your dinner portion and have the leftovers for lunch the following day. On a less-organised day, simply serve your meal on a bed of raw baby spinach and throw a few carrot sticks on the side of the plate. To increase your intake of raw veggies, try juicing (ideally cold-pressed). You can use carrot, celery or beetroot (beet) as a base, adding ingredients like spinach, mint, parsley, ginger and lemon. Smoothies are also an ideal way to boost your raw veggie intake.

FRUIT Aim for a maximum of two pieces of fruit daily. While fruit contains lots of nutrients and fresh enzymes, it also contains high levels of fructose, which can affect blood-sugar levels and may delay ovulation in people with insulin resistance. Be sure to include fruit that is dried, juiced or blended in your daily serves. Try to balance fruit with protein and 'good' fats to ensure a slower release of sugar and energy and avoid the after-sugar slump. Fruit is often eaten in excess because it is so readily available and requires minimal preparation. Chopping up carrots, cucumber, celery, capsicum (pepper) and cherry tomatoes and keeping them in an airtight container in the fridge is a great way to reduce excess fruit consumption and boost your raw veggie intake.

The best fruits to include for balanced hormones are the low glycaemic index (GI) fruits. Low GI foods allow for a longer, more sustained increase in blood sugar, avoiding the spike-and-crash reaction common with high GI foods. Examples of low GI fruits include berries, cherries, pomegranates and plums. Pomegranate has been shown to block the enzyme that coverts fat to oestrogen, making it a powerful food to help balance oestrogen levels in the body.

DRINKS

PURIFIED WATER Water is essential for energy and health and yet so many people I see in my clinic are chronically dehydrated. I often remind them that they need to consider water as their free supplement. If I was to sell them the amount of water they needed to drink before their next appointment, they would divide it up and drink it daily, yet they almost always forget. Many of us don't recognise when we are thirsty or mistake the feeling for hunger. Many women also restrict their water intake to avoid having to go to the bathroom multiple times per day; this is a terrible reason not to drink water! When you are chronically dehydrated, the bladder will shrink and result in frequent urination when you do increase your fluid intake. Stick with it: your bladder capacity will increase as your body gets used to better levels of hydration.

The type of water you drink is probably more important than you think and the best type is filtered tap water. Many people drink only bottled water which may contain hormonally harmful chemicals when they leach from the plastic bottle. Even BPA-free bottles may still contain other forms of plastics and endocrine disruptors. If you need to buy a disposable water bottle, use it once only and try to avoid leaving it in the sun, which can increases the rate of chemicals leaching into the water.

Unfiltered water may contain contaminants such as fertilisers, pesticides and chlorine, which have been linked to unwanted health effects and are also potential hormone disruptors.

A simple and reasonably cost-effective way to reduce contaminants is to invest in a good-quality water filter. These can be installed under the sink, or alternatively a benchtop ceramic filter is also fantastic. Do not store the filtered water in a plastic jug or plastic water bottles. Glass or stainless-steel water bottles and jugs are best.

You should be aiming to drink around 30 ml (1 fl oz) of water per day for every kilogram (2 lb 4 oz) of body weight — around 2 litres (70 fl oz) if you weigh 70 kilograms (155 pounds). You will also need to increase intake when exercising.

YOU SHOULD BE AIMING TO DRINK AROUND 30 ML (1 FL OZ) OF WATER FOR EVERY KILOGRAM (2 LB 4 OZ) OF BODY WEIGHT.

SMOOTHIES AND JUICES Both of these types of drinks can be nutritious when they contain wholefoods and no sugary yoghurts or ice cream, and when you drink them in moderation. The main difference between smoothies and juices is that the juicing process extracts water, vitamins and minerals from the fruit or vegetables, leaving the pulp or fibre behind. Smoothies, on the other hand, contain the whole fruit or vegetable: whatever you put into the blender is consumed in the end product.

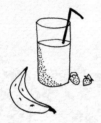

Juicing, especially if the juice is mostly vegetables and leafy greens, can be a nutrient boost and help deliver essential vitamins and minerals in an easily absorbed form. It is ideal to follow the juice with a good-quality fat and protein snack to promote blood-sugar balance. (Try a small handful of nuts and seeds.) The problem with juicing is that large amounts of fructose-containing fruit and vegetables are needed to make just one cup of juice: more than most people would consume in a meal. Without fibre to slow it down, the fructose is rapidly absorbed, which disrupts blood-sugar levels and can lead to fatigue and overeating.

Smoothies are nutrient-dense and, when you start adding vegetables and leafy greens, they are an easy and tasty way to seriously boost your vegetable intake. It is a good idea to lay all the ingredients out before blending, so that you can be sure that what you are about to consume is an appropriate amount of food. Start out with fruity smoothies with an appealing taste and then slowly add vegetables and superfoods, while reducing the amount of fruit. As with any meal or snack, a smoothie should contain three key ingredients: a source of protein (nuts, seeds, tahini, yoghurt, bone broth); a source of 'good' fats (avocado, nuts, seeds, coconut oil); and vegetables (leafy greens, celery, cucumber, carrot, mint, in addition to fruit). If you need to add liquid, try milk, nut milk, coconut milk or filtered water. As you become more advanced in your smoothie-making you can start playing with nutrient-dense foods such as bee pollen, hemp seeds, collagen, spirulina, mesquite, acai and chlorella.

Green smoothies provide an easily absorbed form of essential folate and calcium, keep energy levels high and blood-sugar levels low. They are an easy breakfast option that doesn't include wheat, grains, added sugars or excess dairy. Mint is a great addition as its strong flavour can disguise the more bitter vegetable tastes. Another secret ingredient in delicious green smoothies is frozen mango. Be sure to make extra in the morning and keep leftovers in a screw-top jar in the fridge to enjoy as a snack in the afternoon.

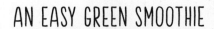

AN EASY GREEN SMOOTHIE

Combine frozen mango, frozen
banana, avocado, celery, baby spinach,
chia seeds, mint and filtered water.
You can start the day knowing that
you have had four different green
vegetables before 8am!

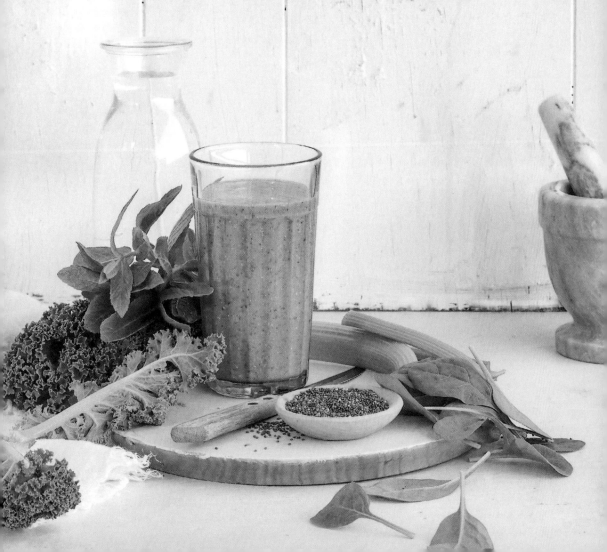

⇒ Herbal Teas ⇐

Herbal teas are a great way to increase your daily fluid intake, especially during the winter months when water intake usually decreases. Always check the ingredient list to ensure the tea does not contain added flavours, sugars or colours. Herbal teas should contain only the herbs.

There are several types of herbal teas that can help to optimise hormonal health. These can support liver function, digestion, stress management and hormonal balance.

Most herbals in these teas have a long history of use as natural medicines. The herbal teas listed here are safe to self-prescribe; however, you should check with a naturopath before using them in higher doses or taking them as tablets or tinctures.

LIVER SUPPORT:

ST MARY'S THISTLE is used for its liver-healing properties and to protect and restore liver cells while promoting healthy liver function. St Mary's thistle is also an anti-inflammatory and antioxidant. St Mary's thistle tea can be consumed daily and is a great support for conditions such as endometriosis, recurrent headaches and premenstrual nausea.

DANDELION ROOT has a long history of culinary and medicinal use, and helps to promote healthy liver function. It also acts as a diuretic. Think of dandelion root as a tea that can spring-clean the body. Dandelion root stimulates digestive juices, reduces inflammation, and is an antioxidant. It helps to clear the body of excess oestrogen and other hormones that may contribute to premenstrual symptoms including low energy, mood swings, hot flushes, bloating, and breast tenderness.

NETTLE LEAF contains a range of minerals such as iron, potassium and silica. Nettle leaf is also thought to reduce excessive menstrual bleeding as well as fluid retention and inflammation. Nettle has anti-allergy properties that may help alleviate hayfever symptoms, dermatitis and itchy skin conditions. Nettle leaf tea is my first choice

for reducing hormone-related fluid retention; drink two cups a day for best results.

DIGESTION:

FENNEL SEED Fennel was known as a magical herb in the Middle Ages and is thought to reduce painful stomach cramps and spasms and calm digestive upsets. Fennel seed tea is a great way to reduce and ease irritable bowel syndrome (IBS) symptoms, colic, flatulence and nausea. Fennel also contains phytoestrogens, which can be helpful for balancing hormones in women with PMS and can improve mood swings and reduce bloating, breast tenderness, hot flushes and fatigue.

LEMON is a wonder fruit of the citrus family as it has so many health benefits! Lemon may aid digestion and boost the metabolism, which promotes liver and kidney function and supports weight loss. Lemon is also very high in vitamin C and other vitamins and minerals that are required for immune-system support. Lemon tea is simply made by squeezing fresh lemon juice into hot water.

CINNAMON is a culinary and medicinal spice that is now known to have blood-sugar regulating qualities. Cinnamon is also an astringent herb that can help to reduce excessive blood flow during menstruation. Cinnamon tea contains cinnamaldehyde, which assists in correcting hormonal imbalances due to its ability to reduce testosterone and increase progesterone. Cinnamon is a useful herb to use for treating PCOS, due to its dual actions on hormonal balance and improving insulin resistance[33].

STRESS SUPPORT:

WITHANIA, also known as ashwaganda, may help the body adapt to stress and change. It is used to calm the nervous system and support mood regulation, reduce inflammation, assist with restful sleep, improve immune-system function and improve cognition. Withania assists hormonal balance by reducing the stress hormone cortisol, which is responsible for increasing oestrogen levels and disrupting hormonal balance.

CHAMOMILE has been used medicinally since Egyptian times and is often used for reducing inflammation, calming and soothing digestive upsets. Chamomile tea is great for relieving premenstrual symptoms such as bloating, painful cramps and irritability. Chamomile tea can also help to reduce anxiety and may help to promote a restful sleep.

LICORICE Licorice root has been used medicinally since prehistoric times to reduce inflammation, protect and soothe sore throats and protect against bacteria and viruses. Licorice tea contains phytoestrogens, which assist in correcting hormonal imbalances, as well as reducing exhaustion, mood swings, irritability, hot flushes, bloating and breast tenderness. Licorice and peony in combination are also known for their hormonal balancing effects and are often used to manage PCOS and infertility. Licorice can be used during times of stress due to its ability to slow down cortisol breakdown. Chronic stress contributes to cortisol depletion, which can lead to an altered stress response where the body is unable to deal with stress in a healthy way. Licorice tea is also used for its immune and anti-inflammatory actions in autoimmune conditions.

HORMONAL BALANCE:

SPEARMINT, from the mint family, is a well-loved culinary and medicinal herb that can be used for reducing stomach cramps, calming and soothing digestive upsets and relieving nausea. Spearmint also contains essential oils that protect against bacteria, and can help to clear and soothe congested airways. Studies have shown spearmint is able to reduce excess androgens such as testosterone, making it useful for conditions such as PCOS, acne and excess body hair. Drink two to three cups daily for this anti-androgenic effect[34].

CHASTE TREE (*Vitex agnus castus*) may have the ability to increase progesterone and inhibit prolactin. It is excellent for women suffering from oestrogen dominance or progesterone deficiency. Chaste tree can help to regulate menstrual cycle length in addition to reducing PMS, breast tenderness, fluid retention, headaches, bloating, anger and irritation. It's advisable to use chaste tree under the supervision of a naturopath[35].

WHITE PEONY is commonly used in traditional herbal medicine for women's reproductive health purposes. White peony works on several levels: as a muscle relaxant, which reduces painful cramps; as an oestrogen modulator, which balances excess oestrogens and androgens; and to reduce inflammation and improve mood. White peony has fabulous hormonal balancing abilities and can assist women suffering from oestrogen dominance, painful periods, irregular periods, heavy periods, endometriosis, uterine fibroids, PCOS, excess body hair, acne and infertility. Avoid during pregnancy and when breastfeeding.

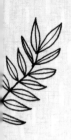

SOMETIMES (BUT NOT VERY OFTEN) FOODS

SUGAR

Refined sugar has been implicated in leaching important nutrients from the body, disrupting healthy gut bacteria, and creating and exacerbating inflammation, as well as affecting stress, mood and energy levels. Excessive refined sugar intake can create inflammation, which is an issue for those with endometriosis, painful periods, backache, acne and nausea[36].

Many women notice that when they have a month with more sugar (and caffeine and alcohol) in their diet, their menstrual and premenstrual symptoms seem to be worse. To check this out for yourself, try going without added sugar for a month. This means avoiding fruit juices, cakes, biscuits, soft drinks, processed foods and even honey. You may be surprised to know that things like white bread and breakfast cereals contain a lot of sugar!

I recommend that you check the ingredient list of packaged foods and avoid added sugar. Try to also minimise the use of natural sugars such as coconut sugar and maple syrup, which contain some beneficial nutrients but are still loaded with saccharides.

It is generally best not to replace processed sugar with a multitude of other sweeteners such as rice malt syrup, stevia, xylitol or dried fruit. These alternatives can be great for the occasional treat, but using them regularly will only keep the sweetness addiction going. If you do indulge in a sweet treat, be mindful: choose something you really like, sit down and enjoy the pleasure it brings.

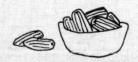

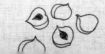

IS SUGAR SO BAD?

Sugar in the blood causes the release of a hormone called insulin, which is closely connected to other hormones in the body including oestrogen and testosterone. Insulin levels in the blood spike after a high-sugar meal and lower the level of an important protein called sex hormone binding globulin (SHBG), which binds to hormones to allow their excretion from the body. Insulin also increases the production of testosterone, which is then converted into even more oestrogen by fatty tissue in the body. When a woman has polycystic ovarian syndrome (PCOS) or her insulin levels are consistently high, insulin resistance can occur, affecting ovulation and implantation. Insulin resistance may also be a precursor to diabetes, so check with your GP if you are worried.

Excess sugar intake is also linked to increased cortisol production. After the sugar high, blood-sugar levels drop, which stimulates the adrenal glands to secrete cortisol and adrenaline to get our energy levels and mood back to normal. When excess cortisol is produced, progesterone production is compromised. The result of all this is oestrogen excess that can lead to irritability, insomnia, anxiety and negative menstrual symptoms.

ALCOHOL

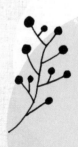

Alcohol has been shown to disrupt normal menstrual cycling, contribute to lack of ovulation and infertility and has been associated with early menopause[37]. A study looked at healthy women who drank small amounts of alcohol (social drinkers) and found that a substantial portion of them stopped cycling normally and became temporarily infertile[38]. I advise women not to consume more than two or three glasses of wine or spirits a week. If you are trying to conceive, I always suggest that you avoid alcohol altogether for three months prior to attempting conception (this goes for both partners).

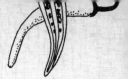

COFFEE

Caffeine is highly addictive, inflammatory and acidic. Coffee can worsen premenstrual symptoms, increase period pain and exacerbate anxiety. Modern society has a huge reliance on coffee and drinking several cups per day is considered normal. If you really love your coffee, try to stick to just one a day. For those trying to conceive, I recommend avoiding caffeine for at least two months before attempting conception, as caffeine has been implicated in fertility, pregnancy and fetal health problems including miscarriage[39]. Decaffeinated coffee is slightly better but still not recommended for daily intake as it may be linked to inflammation. Choose water-decaffeinated coffee if possible, as many coffee roasters use chemical solvents during processing.

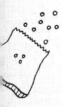

GRAINS

This is the one major food group that does not fall under the categories of protein, 'good' fats or something fresh. Grains include wheat, rye, barley, corn, spelt, kamut (Khorasan wheat), rice, oats, pseudo-grains such as quinoa, amaranth and buckwheat, and foods containing them and their byproducts, such as bread, pasta, cereal and crackers. Minimising or excluding grains allows room for more nutrient-dense foods in your diet. If you do eat grains, they should be an accompaniment to your meal, not the basis of it. Aim for a maximum of one serve per day. Try to choose nutrient-dense grains and pseudo-grains such as buckwheat, quinoa, teff and wild or brown rice. If you don't feel satisfied after a grain-free meal, try to bump up the 'good' fats or add some starchy veggies such as sweet potato and pumpkin.

SHOULD I BE AVOIDING GRAINS?

Grains should probably be avoided if you have an autoimmune condition, inflammatory disease, thyroid disease, polycystic ovarian syndrome (PCOS), insulin resistance or are not ovulating regularly. Consider talking to a naturopath or nutritionist about trying a grain-free diet if you suffer from ongoing fatigue, digestive bloating or allergies. For others, it's a good idea generally to avoid processed grains that have been refined and look for more nutritious options, such as quinoa or wild rice.

FREQUENTLY ASKED QUESTIONS

ARE COCONUTS GOOD OR BAD FOR YOU?

Coconuts are a rich source of electrolytes, which are good for muscle function and hydration. They are loaded with fibre to help keep you full for longer and assist in bowel function. They are also rich in lauric acid, which is only found in coconuts and breast milk. Lauric acid is a medium-chain fatty acid that helps to promote bowel health and enhance immunity. It also possesses antibacterial and antiviral properties. Coconut oil is a really stable fat that doesn't oxidise when heated, making it great for cooking.

When buying coconut cream or milk choose one that is 100 per cent coconut. You can freeze it in icetrays and use it as needed, diluted with water to make your own coconut dairy substitute. Tinned coconut milk has the downside that the tins could contain BPA in the lining, although some manufacturers now use BPA-free tins.

Coconut water is a popular drink and is full of electrolytes, although it contains around a teaspoon of sugar in each cup, so use it in moderation as a treat.

Make your own coconut milk

Line a sieve with muslin (cheesecloth) and set it over a large bowl. Blend 2 cups of coconut flakes with 4 cups of hot water and pour it through the lined sieve. Discard the solids and transfer the liquid to an airtight container or bottle. Add ½ teaspoon of vanilla extract to sweeten if desired. Store in a glass bottle in the fridge for up to three days. Shake before serving.

IS SOY GOOD OR BAD?

Commercially grown soy is often grown using pesticides. Soy also contains phytoestrogens (plant oestrogens), which can affect hormonal balance and health. These phytoestrogens are much milder than environmental oestrogens found in plastics and pesticides, and are also found in common foods such as garlic, lentils, cabbages, dairy and meat. While phytoestrogens can help hormonal balance, excessive consumption of soy products can actually suppress menstruation and cause fertility issues.

Soy is considered to be an antinutrient (blocking the absorption of other essential nutrients) and may inhibit thyroid hormone production in some women. As an antinutrient, soy can inhibit the absorption of essential nutrients and minerals. I would recommend generally

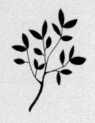

avoiding soy products, in particular more processed ones such as tofu and soy milk. Fermented or whole soy products such as tamari, tempeh, miso and edamame beans can be consumed in moderation.

SHOULD I GIVE UP BREAD?

Some people find bread difficult to digest and it can also contain unwanted ingredients such as sugars and preservatives. When bread is traditionally prepared via soaking and fermenting, the nutrients become more available for digestion. Commercial breads often contain high levels of phytic acid, which reduces the absorption of minerals including calcium, magnesium, zinc, copper and iron.

In many countries, synthetic folic acid (sometimes incorrectly called folate) is added to commercial breads. This fortification is fine for people who are able to absorb synthetic folic acid, but it is not so good for those who have a polymorphism on the gene that is responsible for the metabolism and absorption of folate. These people may not be able to metabolise synthetic folic acid and may need supplementation with an activated form of folate called 5-methyltetrahydrafolate (also known as L-methylfolate or 5–MTHF)[40]. If you eat bread, look for a traditionally prepared loaf from a local bakery with minimal ingredients, such as a spelt sourdough, sprouted loaf or a gluten-free option from a wholefoods store or bakery.

LOOK FOR A TRADITIONALLY PREPARED LOAF FROM A LOCAL BAKERY WITH MINIMAL INGREDIENTS, SUCH AS A SPELT SOURDOUGH.

CAN I HAVE GLUTEN?

Gluten is the major protein found in wheat, rye, barley, spelt, kamut (Khorosan wheat) and oats. Gluten is a protein that can be quite difficult to digest and inflammatory for some people; while others have coeliac disease, which is a condition in which the immune system reacts abnormally to gluten, causing bowel damage, inflammation and impaired nutrient absorption. Other people find that they have a sensitivity to gluten that can cause fatigue, bloating and other digestive symptoms.

Undiagnosed coeliac disease and gluten intolerance can be a contributing factor in infertility and miscarriage. Gluten intolerance and coeliac disease can be tested by your doctor; if you think you might be gluten intolerant or coeliac it's important to be tested before you cut gluten out of your diet.

Gluten is also particularly unfriendly for those with thyroid disorders or autoimmune dieases. A part of the gluten molecule closely resembles thyroid tissue and stimulates an immune response that causes the body to attack the thyroid. Your doctor or naturopath will be able to advise on whether you need to cut down or eliminate gluten if this is the case.

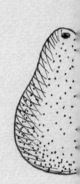

It is worth trying a gluten-free diet for two months if you suffer from period pain, joint aches, headaches, fatigue, foggy thinking, digestive disturbance, mood disorders or have been diagnosed by a doctor with an elevated level of Natural Killer Cells (these are related to your immune system). After the two months is up, assess your symptoms. If you don't have a problem with gluten, you can still choose to use it sparingly in your diet and remember to keep loading up on vegetables.

DO I REALLY NEED SEVEN TYPES OF VEGETABLES EVERY DAY?

Aiming for seven types of vegetables (around four or five cups uncooked) ensures that you will eat a wide variety of nutrients every day. You can include things like garlic and herbs in the seven types, although they won't do much to help you get up to four or five cups, so make sure that you bulk out what you are eating by including vegetables with most meals. For the purposes of this section, you can count salad vegetables that are technically classified as fruits — such as cucumber, tomato and avocado — in your vegetable tally.

Try to get a good mix of raw (salad) and cooked vegetables. While salads are great, they tend to not include important hormone-friendly vegetables such as broccoli, cauliflower, asparagus and brussels sprouts. If you are minimising grains, make sure you include some starchy veggies for energy and satiety. Good choices are baked pumpkin (squash) and sweet potato.

If you are eating leftovers from dinner as your lunch (an excellent idea), it is easier to reach the recommended vegetable intake. Add some spinach and avocado to your morning eggs, snack on carrot and celery with hummus, and all of a sudden it's not hard to reach the target of seven types a day.

NUTRITION FOR DIFFERENT TIMES IN YOUR CYCLE

DURING YOUR PERIOD (Day 1 until the end of bleeding)

This is a time when many women feel hormonally imbalanced, which can result in feeling tired, crampy, bloated and moody. Remember to be kind to yourself and, if you need a treat or indulgence, try a nutritious option such as Bliss balls (see page 204).

During this stage, blood loss will require lots of iron- and vitamin C-rich foods to restore your depleted stores. Excellent food sources of iron include red meat, asparagus, silverbeet (Swiss chard), spinach, thyme, turmeric and cumin seeds. Vitamin C helps to increase the absorption of iron and keep the blood vessels strong: good choices include red capsicum (peppers), broccoli, strawberries, kiwifruit, tomatoes and citrus.

Liver-friendly foods for hormonal support are essential during this time. Bulk up on broccoli, cauliflower, asparagus, brussels sprouts, garlic, cabbage and spinach while avoiding caffeine, sugar and alcohol: these will only add to the load your liver has to process, and we need it in top working condition! Opt for organically grown fruit and veg if you can.

Anti-inflammatory foods can help to reduce pain and inflammation. Increase your intake of oily fish such as wild-caught salmon and sardines, add turmeric and ginger to smoothies, curries and soups (sprinkle grated turmeric and ginger into your morning omelette for an easy boost) and increase your intake of berries and cherries when in season.

Make sure you are drinking lots of fluids (water and herbal tea… not coffee!) to reduce clotting and minimise headaches and fatigue. Try our delicious Turmeric chai (see page 231) as an indulgent option.

turmeric

PREPARING FOR OVULATION: THE FOLLICULAR PHASE

After your period is over, you are usually feeling pretty good as oestrogen levels rise in preparation for ovulation. If you are trying to conceive, load up on B vitamins, zinc and vitamin C to support the release of an egg and promote implantation.

Avoid inflammatory foods, such as caffeine, sugar, processed grains and alcohol, which can make your cervical mucus hostile to sperm. Increase your intake of leafy greens, cruciferous vegetables and purified water.

'Good' fats are essential for hormone production, so adding avocado, wild-caught salmon, sardines, walnuts, chia seeds, coconut oil and almond milk to your diet is a great idea. Avoid processed fats, fried foods and trans fats. Ask a naturopath about supplementing your diet with omega-3 essential fatty acids.

Boost your cervical mucus production by increasing your intake of calcium-rich foods such as full-fat Greek-style yoghurt, unhulled tahini, hummus, chia seeds, almonds, figs, sardines, spinach, broccoli, parsley and watercress.

INCREASE YOUR INTAKE OF LEAFY GREENS, CRUCIFEROUS VEGETABLES AND PURIFIED WATER.

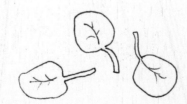

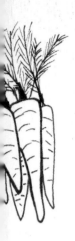

THE LUTEAL PHASE (usually around 14 days)

The first half of this phase is when oestrogen declines and your body starts increasing progesterone production. Exercise regularly and try to get seven to nine hours of good-quality sleep per night. Increase progesterone-friendly foods such as those containing vitamin B6, magnesium, zinc and vitamin C.

Increasing your intake of leafy greens and orange vegetables, such as carrots, pumpkins (squash) and sweet potato, will balance hormones and support cell division and implantation. Try adding fresh pineapple to a green smoothie to benefit from the bromelians in pineapple that may help to support implantation, reduce inflammation in the gut and taste great as well!

Reduce salt in your diet to ease fluid retention, and increase your intake of vegetables using some of the tips on page 114.

The second half of the luteal phase is when many women will begin to experience premenstrual stress (or the anxiety and anticipation of waiting to do a pregnancy test). Practise lots of self care during this week by not overcommitting yourself. Go for regular walks, take a yoga class or spend some time outside in the sun: anything that helps you feel connected and calm and that supports your body in a healthy way.

This is the time to avoid sugar, caffeine and alcohol to keep your blood-sugar levels as stable as possible. Eat protein with each meal, snack when you need to and make sure that you don't leave long gaps between meals.

Foods that are warm, well-cooked, soaked, stewed, steamed or sprouted can be great for nourishing your body and soul at this time. Herbal teas are great between and after meals: choose from cinnamon, fennel, licorice, nettle, peppermint, ginger and chamomile.

Avoid salads (especially uncooked leaves), hard and raw fruits (particularly apples), whole nuts and undercooked vegetables.

As always it is important to drink lots of water: aim for your urine to be mostly clear.

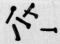

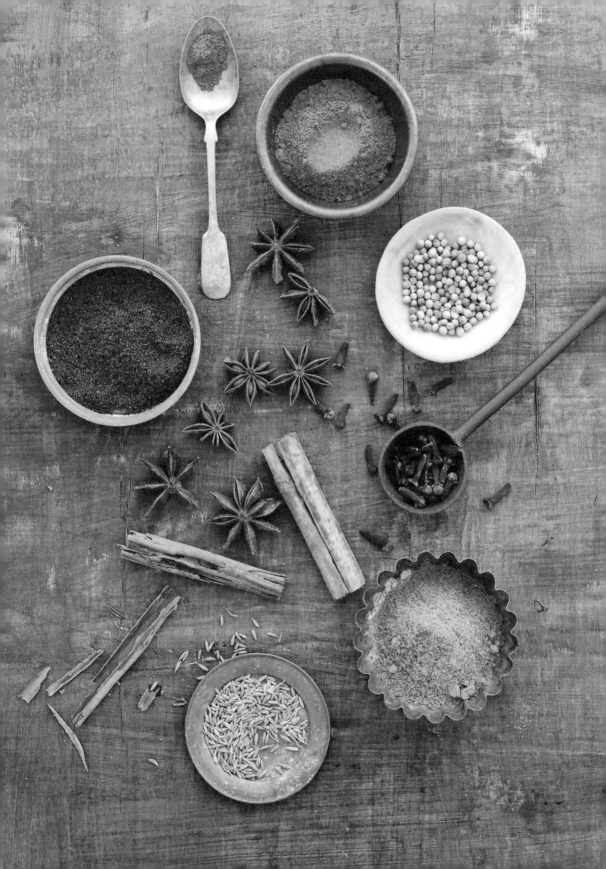

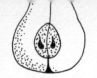

UNDERSTANDING SUPPLEMENTS

While most of us would prefer to obtain all our nutrients from the food we eat, the reality is that sometimes our needs are greater than what we can eat or absorb from our diet. This may be due to poor nutrient quality in food, too many processed foods, a lack of vital nutrients in our soil or an increased need for certain nutrients due to stress or health conditions. Nutritional supplements can be used to correct nutrient deficiencies or can be used in therapeutic doses to manage and treat certain conditions.

It is advisable to have a naturopath prescribe supplements specifically for you to ensure you are taking everything you need (and nothing you don't); to indicate how long you should take the supplement for; and also to ensure that there are no contraindications. Always mention any supplements you are taking to your doctor to make sure there are no conflicts with prescription medicines.

Some common supplements that your naturopath might prescribe are listed here. For more detailed information, see page 232.

SUPPLEMENT	EFFECT	WHO MIGHT NEED IT?
FISH OILS	anti-inflammatory	people who do not eat fish, those suffering from inflammation, pain or auto-immune diseases
ZINC	regulates and supports cycles, blocks excess androgens	women with PCOS and women wanting to conceive, women taking the contraceptive pill
CoQ10 (Coenzyme Q)	energy production, antioxidant	women wanting to conceive, especially over the age of 35 and those undergoing IVF treatment
NAC (N-acetyl cysteine)	antioxidant, anti-inflammatory	women with endometriosis or PCOS and those wanting to conceive
LIPOIC ACID	antioxidant	women with PCOS and/or those wanting to conceive
IODINE	used to make thyroid hormones	requirements are increased during pregnancy

VITAMIN D	essential for progesterone production, immunity, bone health and healthy mood	people who spend little time in the sun and those who cover exposed skin with sunscreen or clothes; people with dark skin may also require vitamin D supplementation
IRON	essential for energy and immune function and important in pregnancy	women who experience heavy menstrual blood loss, vegetarians and vegans may benefit from iron supplementation
PROBIOTICS	maintain healthy intestinal bacteria	people with a low intake of fibre, those who have been on antibiotics and those with chronic low immunity or digestive issues
VITAMIN E	antioxidant and anti-inflammatory	women with oestrogen deficiency, thin uterine lining or scanty bleeds in addition to older women trying to conceive and those undergoing IVF
VITAMIN C	antioxidant, immune stimulant	people with low immune function (recurrent colds and flu), those who consume minimal fresh fruit and vegetables, those experiencing stress or with low progesterone
CALCIUM	essential for healthy bones	increase at menopause to prevent osteoporosis; also those with hypothalamic amenorrhoea
MAGNESIUM	relax muscles and calm the nervous system	those experiencing muscle cramps, poor sleep, fatigue and relative progesterone deficiency
VITAMIN B6	progesterone production, healthy mood, PMS	women with symptoms of PMS such as fluid retention, cramping, anxiety, depression, insomnia
VITAMIN B12	energy production, healthy mood, helps to make DNA, essential for healthy ovulation and fertility	vegetarians and vegans, women with heavy periods and those trying to conceive
FOLATE	essential during pregnancy and for at least three months prior to conception	those with a genetic defect in folate metabolism may require folate supplementation in addition to women wanting to conceive
CHROMIUM	helps control blood-sugar levels as well as the metabolism of protein and fat	those with insulin resistance and sugar cravings or those who consume high amounts of carbohydrate foods
INOSITOL	promotes ovulation and helps with insulin resistance	those with PCOS, hypothyroidism, experiencing stress, low mood or anxiety
SELENIUM	supports thyroid health	selenium is very low in Australian soil, which means that deficiency is common
DiINOLYMETHANE (DIM) / INDOLE-3-CARBINOL (I-3-C)	may reduce the risk of breast and cervical cancer	women with endometriosis and oestrogen excess, women with family history of breast or cervical cancer may also benefit

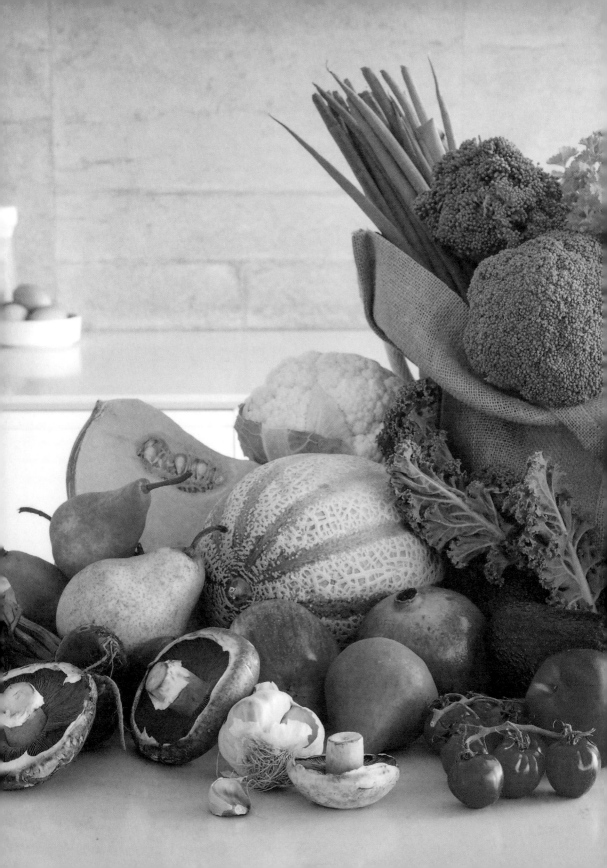

Food Preparation and Planning

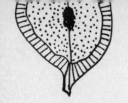

FOOD PREPARATION
and *planning*

When you first start focusing on nutrition and meal planning, it can feel like a big effort and something that takes up valuable time; however, it can become something you incorporate into your routine.

The trick is to think ahead. When you are chopping vegetables for dinner, chop some extra to munch on the following day. While you are waiting for dinner to cook, boil some eggs for breakfast in the morning. This way, little extra time for food prep is required; you are just making the most of time you already have. Always cook an extra portion of dinner and pop it straight into your lunch box as you are serving, ready to take to work the following day. Putting it straight into the lunch box and into the fridge stops anyone from eating your lunch as their second helping!

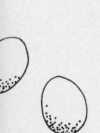

Make a rough plan of what you will be eating over the next couple of days for breakfast, morning snack, lunch, afternoon snack and dinner. You might be surprised at how much a rough plan (I just use the notes app on my smartphone) helps to keep you on track. Make sure you write down your meals, buy the ingredients or organise an online delivery so the ingredients are all in your fridge when you want them.

GETTING ORGANISED

★ **The more you make your favourite recipes, the easier and quicker the prep becomes.** For example, once you've made our banana bread (see page 163) a few times, you'll find it can be made by the time the oven has heated up and you are ready to bake!

★ **Buy in bulk.** Go to a bulk wholefoods store or trusted website and stock up. You can often take your own containers to places like these, then not only are you helping eliminate waste, you will be one step ahead on the organisation front. Winning!

★ **Implement a regular toasting time.** Turn your oven on and load up a bunch of trays with nuts and seeds. Nuts and seeds all vary in toasting times and can easily burn at the edges so do keep a sharp eye on them.

★ **Soak a big batch of chickpeas and other legumes.** Before you go to bed, pop them in a bowl, cover with water and leave overnight. Have your storage containers or resealable plastic bags ready. In the morning, simply drain and store in the freezer until you are ready to use them.

★ Grab some resealable plastic bags and **make up a bunch of smoothie ingredient bags** for the freezer. When you need to make a smoothie, just pop them in the blender with your choice of milk or water.

★ To ensure a nutritious diet, **start moving away from packaged and ready-made meals** and takeaway and start cooking at home.

★ **Make your own stock or broth.** When you have the ingredients in the fridge and a slow cooker, take five minutes to put them all in the slow cooker in the evening. Turn it on to the low setting and the next morning you have a ready-made nutritious stock ready to strain and use.

★ Pop any leftover broccoli or cauliflower stems, kale leaves and other **vegetable offcuts into a bag or container in the freezer** ready for soup or stock making.

★ On the weekend, **make up a few dressings** so that they are ready for using on salads during the week.

★ **Love your leftovers.** Try to cook at least one extra serving of each meal, that way you have the next day's lunch packed up and ready to go.

★ **Make up a few batches of buckwheat crepes** (see page 182). They can be stored in the freezer and are great for breakfast with fruit or to wrap up a salad for lunch.

★ **Poach a few pieces of chicken breast** on the weekend (see page 211) and shred the meat, ready to be used in wraps or on crackers.

NUTRITIOUS MEAL SUGGESTIONS

BREAKFAST

Start the day with a nutritious breakfast. Prepare the ingredients as much as you can before bed to ensure a speedy start.

Chia pudding or porridge (see page 170)

Omelette with greens and goat's cheese

Smoothie (try the Berry ripe smoothie on page 178)

Boiled eggs with avocado, spinach and pesto (or try the Egg stack with pesto on page 166)

Greek yoghurt with linseed, sunflower seed and almond meal (LSA) and berries (see page 156)

DRINKS

Water is your free supplement! It increases energy, helps maintain healthy body weight, increases cervical mucus and supports healthy blood flow that carries nutrients around your body. Set an alarm to remember to drink water and aim for around 2 litres (70 fl oz/8 cups) every day. Herbal teas count in your water intake.

LUNCH

The easiest thing to do is to make an extra serving of dinner and pack it up for lunch the following day. Otherwise try chicken, pumpkin (squash), avocado, pesto and mixed leaf salad; salads or soups from the recipe section; or frittata and salad. Buckwheat crepes (see page 182) with salmon can also be eaten at lunch time. If you need to buy takeaway, try these:

Sashimi salad with miso soup

Mexican burrito bowl

A big salad with chicken or salmon

Falafel bowl with hummus and tabouleh

Grilled fish and salad

Asian stir-fried vegetables with chicken, beef or lamb

Pho soup with extra green veggies

Second breakfast: eggs with avocado, haloumi, fresh herbs and spinach

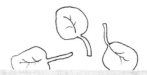

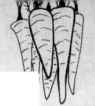

DINNER

Choose a protein (meat, chicken, fish, eggs or legumes) and add as many vegetables as you can. Use fresh herbs and spices for taste and always drizzle a little olive oil or coconut oil over steamed vegetables for taste and satisfaction. If you are hungry, add baked root vegetables or mashed sweet potato and pumpkin (squash), cauliflower, quinoa or kelp noodles. Dinner options could be:

Fish with steamed vegetables, salad or ratatouille

Baked or roast meat with a big serving of salad or steamed vegetables

Stir-fried vegetables with nuts, sesame and sunflower seeds, pine nuts and tempeh

Chickpea or lentil patties served with vegetables and salad

Roast chicken with roasted carrot, onion, sweet potato and steamed greens

Vegetable frittata with salad

Marinated organic chicken skewers with steamed pumpkin and green vegetables

SNACKS

Prepare snacks in advance to save time! On Sunday and Wednesday nights I try to prepare enough snacks to last three days. Examples include:

Boiled eggs

Nuts and seeds

Trail mix

Leftover smoothie

Chia pudding (see page 228)

Apple with almond butter

Hummus and carrot, celery or cucumber sticks

Miso soup

Bliss balls (see page 204)

Nutty banana bread (see page 163)

Cheese and cucumber

Greek yoghurt with LSA and berries

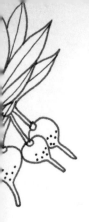

SHOPPING

READING LABELS

Many food labels are designed to convince the consumer that the product is a healthy choice. Claims of 'organic', 'natural', 'sugar-free', 'fat-free', 'added vitamins', 'gluten-free' and 'low GI' are often unsubstantiated and mean nothing. Sometimes the food is in brown earthy-looking packaging to make the buyer feel that they are choosing a natural and nutritious product.

When shopping, it is important to be very aware of these marketing techniques: ignore the hype and go straight to the ingredient list. Australian laws require every ingredient to be listed; if that's not the case in your country you need to be even more vigilant. If you're not sure what's in the packaged food you're buying, the following shopping guide will give you some more information to help you make wise choices.

ADDED SUGARS

If sugar is an ingredient, in any form, I'd advise you to put the product back on the shelf. The tricky part is that added sugar is hiding in a large percentage of packaged foods. There are at least 60 different names for sugar (saccharides) that may be listed on labels, including sucrose, glucose, high-fructose corn syrup, barley malt, dextrose, maltose, fructose, evaporated cane juice.

I prefer to avoid all added sugars in food as opposed to looking too much at the quantity of sugar listed on the product nutrition panel, as the panel does not differentiate between added sugar and sugars that occur naturally in foods. I also avoid synthetic sweeteners, such as aspartame, sucralose, saccharin and neotame. If you want an occasional sweet treat, enjoy it and recognise that it is a treat. Watch out for added sugar in products that don't even taste sweet, such as cereals, crackers and yoghurts.

ORGANIC

The only claim that can't be verified by looking at the ingredient list is for organic products. There is no law against products using the word 'organic', so always check for a certification mark from an independent, recognised certifier when you want to buy organic.

GLUTEN FREE

For those who choose or need to eat gluten free, the surge in commercially available gluten-free products can seem like a blessing. Whole supermarket aisles are dedicated to these products; however, I usually recommend you stay well clear of this aisle. While these products may be free of gluten, they are often packed with every other non-gluten, non-food, over-processed ingredient you can think of. There are exceptions to this rule and, if you become an ingredient-list-reading super-sleuth, you may just find a few wholefood products that contain natural ingredients and taste good. When switching to gluten-free, it's best to ditch most processed foods and focus on fresh foods and an abundance of proteins, 'good' fats and fresh fruit and vegetables. All the recipes and meal suggestions in this book just happen to be gluten free, so try some of our recipes.

FOCUS ON CROWDING OUT THE GLUTEN RATHER THAN REPLACING IT WITH OVERPROCESSED ALTERNATIVES.

FATS AND OILS

'Bad' fats are damaging to your hormones and your health and should be avoided. Oils we recommend are coconut oil, olive oil, macadamia oil, organically produced butter and ghee. All seed and vegetable oils should be avoided, including grapeseed oil, rice bran oil, soybean oil, canola oil, corn oil, cottonseed oil, peanut oil, rapeseed oil, safflower oil, sunflower oil and vegetable oil. These oils contain high amounts of omega-6, which is associated with inflammation and inflammatory diseases such as endometriosis, obesity, autoimmune disease, asthma, irritable bowel syndrome, cardiovascular disease and more.

When a product has been processed to become shelf stable, it will usually contain not only seed oils but also the super-damaging trans fats, also known as partially hydrogenated fats.

Low-fat foods are also not recommended due to the extra processing that they go through. Low-fat foods are often full of sugar or other artificial ingredients to make them more tasty, in addition to being less satisfying and making you want more and more of the product.

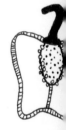

INGREDIENT GLOSSARY

The glossary contains a list of the nutritious wholefoods used in our recipes, with notes on what they are good for, where to find them and how to use them.

ALMOND BUTTER – high in calcium, protein, 'good' fats and fibre. Found in the health-food aisle of most supermarkets or made fresh in some health-food stores. Almond butter can be substituted with other nut or seed butters including cashew, macadamia or sunflower seed. All nut butters should be 100 per cent of the nut or seed and contain no vegetable oil, sugar or other ingredients.

ALMOND MEAL – high in calcium, protein, 'good' fats and fibre. Found in the health-food aisle of most supermarkets, it should contain ground whole almonds with visible flecks of the brown skin. Avoid the blanched almond meal from the baking section. You can make your own meal by grinding almonds in an electric coffee bean grinder. Keep almond meal in the fridge to keep it fresh and prevent the 'good' fats from becoming rancid. Almond meal is a great for baking muffins and pancakes, or adding to porridge.

ALMOND MILK – is a great dairy-free substitute for cow's milk, if it is just made from almonds and water. Be aware that most packaged almond milks and other nut milks contain just two per cent almonds, plus water, sunflower oil, sugar and emulsifiers to keep it all from separating. Making your own almond milk is easy: soak a cup of almonds in water overnight. Drain and peel the almonds. Put them into a blender with 1 litre (35 fl oz/4 cups) of water and blend until smooth. Strain through a piece of muslin (cheesecloth), gently squeezing to allow the milk to collect in a bowl. Store in an airtight glass bottle in the fridge for up to 3 days. Blend again with some vanilla, stevia or a couple of soaked dates to sweeten if needed. Alternatively, fresh almond milk can usually be found in the fridge at your local supermarket or health-food store.

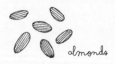

almonds

APPLE CIDER VINEGAR – can be used in salad dressings or diluted with water and consumed before a meal to help with digestion. Look for an unrefined vinegar, which has a cloudy appearance and contains 'the mother' (visible as a cloudy culture of 'good' bacteria in the bottom of the liquid). Apple cider vinegar is thought to boost immunity, promote healthy hair and skin, and may contribute to keeping blood-sugar levels stable. Always swish water around your mouth after consuming, to reduce the impact of the vinegar on your tooth enamel.

APRICOTS, DRIED – high in vitamin C, iron and fibre, they are also high in antioxidants and may help to reduce inflammation. Most dried apricots from supermarkets are treated with sulphur dioxide (220) to extend their shelf life. This preservative will be in the ingredient list so always check before you purchase. Sulphur-free dried apricots will usually be a dark brown colour and are more commonly available from health-food stores. Dried apricots are high in sugar and should be only eaten in moderation, but are a great sweetener to use in baked goods. Remember that two small dried apricot halves are equivalent to one piece of your daily fruit allowance.

BAKING POWDER – helps to fluff up baked goods and is essential for grain-free baking. Baking powder is a combination of bicarbonate of soda (baking soda) and cream of tartar. Look for a brand that is free of aluminium in the baking section of the supermarket.

BRAZIL NUTS – high in protein, 'good' fats and selenium. Just four to five brazil nuts can help you get your daily dose of selenium, which helps support thyroid health and fertility. Look for these nuts in your supermarket or health-food store. As with all nuts and seeds, be sure that they are fresh and keep them in the fridge.

BUCKWHEAT FLOUR – buckwheat is a nutritious grain-like seed that should be avoided when following a grain-free diet, but can otherwise be consumed in moderation. Buckwheat is high in protein, manganese, copper, magnesium and fibre. Buckwheat flour can be found in health-food stores and should be kept in an airtight container in the fridge.

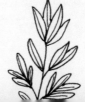

BUTTER – 100 per cent organic butter contains vitamins and is considered hormone friendly. Be careful not to just buy 'butter' from the supermarket and believe that it is pure butter. Butter in tubs will often have added vegetable oils to help it spread easily, so be sure to check the ingredients. If you can find grass-fed butter, that is an even better option. Butter can be used in cooking or for stirring through steamed vegetables.

CACAO – raw cacao powder is full of antioxidants and resveratrol, both of which are great for protecting your ovaries and help to reduce the signs of ageing. Cacao can help boost mood and reduce cardiovascular disease risk, in addition to being full of important minerals. Raw cacao can be found in health-food stores and can be added to smoothies, bliss balls and chia puddings, or try making your own chocolate.

CARAMELISED RED WINE VINEGAR – red wine vinegar is not quite as nutritious as apple cider vinegar and is quite high in histamines, so it's best avoided if you have allergies. The caramelised version does have a little sugar to make it sweet, but if you are not using it too much and don't have any negative reactions then enjoy the taste and use it sparingly.

CHIA SEEDS – these are a true superfood containing loads of omega-3s, antioxidants, fibre, iron, magnesium, calcium and potassium. Not only are these tiny seeds packed full of nutrients, they are also a great source of complete and available protein. The fibre in chia seeds helps with the excretion of hormones from the body and keeps the digestive system moving. Chia seeds have almost no taste, which means they can be added to almost any meal. Aim for at least a tablespoon of chia seeds most days. Keep chia seeds in the fridge to protect the omega-3s.

CHICKEN STOCK – high in protein, zinc, calcium, iron and gut-healing glutamine. Meat stocks or bone broths are ideally made fresh from pasture-fed organic bones. This is important, because you want to make sure that you don't also get any pesticide or chemical residue that has been locked away in the bones of the animal. If you are buying ready-made stock, look for fresh stock that is kept in the fridge section of many butchers or health-food stores and, as usual, check the ingredient list. Avoid powdered stock cubes, which are full of synthetic ingredients.

CHICKPEAS (garbanzo beans) – contain zinc, folate and fibre and are a great way to get some vegetarian protein into your diet. To reduce the presence of nutrient-blocking phytates and improve digestibility, chickpeas should always be soaked overnight before cooking. If you are short on time, you can use tinned chickpeas. Look for a brand that uses BPA-free tins and check the ingredients to avoid any additives. Use chickpeas to make your own hummus or add to salads and casseroles for extra protein and satiety.

CINNAMON – one of my very favourite spices! Cinnamon helps to make things taste sweet, helps to reduce sugar cravings and stabilises blood sugar levels. Ground cinnamon is found in the spices section of the supermarket and can be added liberally to smoothies, baked goods, yoghurt, chia porridge and so much more.

COCONUT, DESICCATED (shredded) – is made from dried coconut meat that has been grated or finely ground. Found in the baking section of the supermarket, desiccated coconut can be used in baked goods, smoothies, porridges and sprinkled over yoghurt or chia puddings.

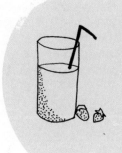

COCONUT FLOUR – a great gluten-free alternative for baking, coconut flour is high in 'good' fats and fibre. Coconut flour is made from ground and dried coconut meat, and is versatile and delicious!

COCONUT MILK – coconut milk is a popular alternative to cow's milk. Unfortunately, most packaged coconut milk also contains vegetable oils, emulsifiers and sugar. I recommend using 100 per cent coconut cream from a BPA-free can and diluting it with water. You can then freeze it in an icetray and pop out the cubes as needed for smoothies, chia puddings and porridges. You can also learn to make your own coconut milk from shredded coconut (see page 123).

COCONUT OIL – this heat-stable oil contains a type of saturated fat called medium-chain fatty acids. These are more easily absorbed than many other types of fats. Coconut oil also contains lauric acid, a type of fat only found in human breast milk and coconuts. Lauric acid is great for the immune system and supports healthy digestion in addition to having antifungal and antibacterial properties. Due to its saturated fat content, coconut oil is not recommended for those watching their cholesterol. It does not oxidise easily at high temperatures, thus making it ideal for cooking on the stovetop, such as when making a stir-fry. The main thing to look for is the virgin, unrefined oil that is produced by pressing raw coconut.

CURRANTS – similar to sultanas but smaller and with a slightly sour taste. They are full of potassium, vitamin B6 and iron and give a great boost of flavour to salads and casseroles. Currants should be eaten in moderation, because like other dried fruits they are quite high in sugar. Look for a brand that doesn't have vegetable oil or sulphur dioxide (220) added as a preservative.

DATES – high in potassium, iron, magnesium and selenium. They are a great source of soluble fibre for good digestive health and can give you a quick energy boost. Dates are great to help sweeten baked goods without using added sugar; however, they are high in fructose. Enjoy in moderation and make sure you count each date into your daily fruit intake. Look for plump fresh dates from a greengrocer and keep in an airtight container for several months.

DUKKAH – a delicious toasted seed and spice blend, dukkah provides a burst of flavour in addition to some 'good' fats, protein and anti-inflammatory spices. Dukkah is available in most supermarkets and specialty stores, or try making your own for a perfect blend. Dukkah is great sprinkled over roast vegetables and salads or combined with oil and used as a marinade for chicken and meat.

FETA – high in protein, calcium and 'good' fats, feta is a traditional Greek cheese usually made from goat's or sheep's milk. This makes feta easier to digest and less inflammatory than traditional cow's milk cheese. Look for an organic brand in the supermarket and consume it in moderation. Feta is a great addition to salads and omelettes or served on a slice of cucumber with a sprinkle of pepper for an easy afternoon snack.

FIG VINO COTTO – made from grape juice concentrate, figs and red wine vinegar. Fig vino cotto is a sweet syrup that blends beautifully with vinegars and sauces and is also used in baking. Fig vino cotto can be found in some supermarkets and specialty grocery stores. It is high in natural sugars and can be used sparingly to provide a rich and delicious taste. Look for a brand that does not contain the preservative sulphur dioxide (220).

FIGS, DRIED – high in calcium, magnesium and iron, figs have about half the sugar and almost double the fibre of dates. Figs are still sweet and should be enjoyed in moderation in baked goods or finely chopped and used in chia puddings and porridges. Dried figs are commonly available in supermarkets and health-food stores.

FISH SAUCE – an Asian flavouring that makes things taste salty and delicious. Sadly, nearly all fish sauce brands contain sugar, preservatives and monosodium glutamate (MSG). Try to find one that only contains two ingredients: fermented anchovies and sea salt. Only a little fish sauce is used at a time and a bottle lasts for a long time, so take the time to source the more nutritious type.

FRUIT, FROZEN – raspberries, blueberries, strawberries, mango, pineapple and even avocado are all now readily available in the freezer section of most supermarkets. This allows us to enjoy these fruits in smoothies and baked goods at a reasonable price, all year round. Most stores offer certified organic frozen fruits, which are highly recommended. I also keep a stash of peeled and chopped frozen bananas to thicken smoothies and make 'ice cream'.

GARLIC POWDER – garlic powder doesn't contain all the benefits of fresh garlic, but is super convenient and tasty. Find it in the herbs and spices section of the supermarket. Check that the ingredients only contain 100 per cent garlic, with no artificial flavours and wheat thickeners. Garlic powder should ideally be organically produced.

GOAT'S CHEESE – rich in calcium, protein and vitamins, goat's cheese has less lactose and is generally easier to digest than cow's milk cheese. Goat's cheese has a distinctive flavour and thus may not be as more-ish as cow's cheese, which helps with portion control! Sprinkle goat's cheese onto salads or into omelettes.

GOJI BERRIES – often referred to as the most nutritionally dense food on Earth. A goji berry is a small, slightly salty dried berry that is not too sweet. They are a great source of vitamins B and C and a potent source of antioxidants. Goji berries are available in health-food stores and make a good snack with nuts and seeds, or they can be chopped up and added to chia puddings, salads and baked goods.

HALOUMI – a delicious salty sheep's cheese that is a great source of calcium, protein and fats. It is found in supermarkets and is the perfect cheese for grilling or barbecuing. Add a squeeze of lemon juice after cooking and add to salads or serve as a side dish.

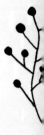

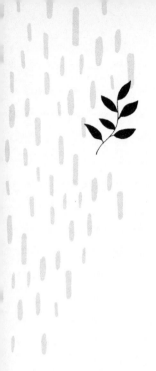

HONEY – high in fructose and glucose, honey should only be consumed in moderation. Many people think that honey can be used freely but it is still high in inflammatory sugar. When buying honey, choose raw, local honey or manuka honey. These types of honey are antibacterial, antifungal, anti-allergy and can help to relieve mouth and throat irritations. A local farmers' market is a good place to find honey. Note that raw honey is not recommended for pregnant women, small children and those with compromised immune systems because it has not been heat treated to remove bacterial and fungal contaminants.

LENTILS – are a great source of folate, iron, magnesium, protein and fibre. They are an alkaline protein source and may help to balance acidity in the body. There are many varieties of lentils, including red, puy, brown and green. Dried lentils are best soaked overnight before cooking to help neutralise any phytates and improve digestibility (red lentils do not need to be soaked). Tinned lentils are available; ideally you should choose a brand that does not use BPA-lined tins.

LINSEEDS (flaxseeds) – the richest plant source of omega-3 fatty acids. They have a pleasant, nutty flavour. Linseeds are quite hard and can be difficult to digest so they are ideally crushed or ground in a coffee grinder before use. Store in the fridge to keep fresh.

LSA – stands for linseed, sunflower seed and almond and comes in the form of blended ground meals. It can be found in the health-food aisle of most supermarkets. LSA is a great source of protein, calcium, 'good' fats and fibre. LSA should be kept in the fridge when you get home to keep the fats fresh and reduce rancidity. Add LSA to smoothies, yoghurt, porridges and baking.

MACADAMIA OIL – has a mild buttery flavour and is great for supporting heart health, lowering triglycerides and stimulating circulation. Macadamia oil is a good substitute for coconut oil in baking and is delicious as a salad dressing.

NAVY/WHITE BEANS – high in folate, protein and manganese, white beans are a great source of cholesterol-lowering fibre and make a delicious vegetarian breakfast or side dish. White beans can be bought from most supermarkets as dried beans that need to be soaked overnight before cooking to improve nutrient availability and reduce potential flatulence. White beans are high in oxalates and should be consumed in moderation by those with kidney stones. Tinned beans are available, but always check for a brand that uses BPA-free tins.

OLIVE OIL, EXTRA VIRGIN – also know as EVOO, olive oil is a healthy fat. Cold-pressed extra virgin olive oil is the best form to look for and should be used at room temperature. Olive oil can be used for baking in the oven as the diffuse heat does not cause it to oxidise. Olive oil can also be drizzled over salads and steamed vegetables and is excellent for creating satiety. Always store olive oil in a dark container in a cool, dry place.

PEANUT BUTTER – a good source of protein and fats, 100 per cent peanut butter can be a delicious snack. Make sure you ditch the processed versions that are loaded with sugar and vegetable oils. Peanuts are not as nutritious as other nuts, so try rotating peanut butter with other nut butters such as almond or cashew.

PEPITAS (pumpkin seeds) – high in zinc, protein and 'good' fats and a top fertility food. Pepitas are a great snack that can be added to trail mix and salads or eaten on their own. As one of the top plant sources of zinc, pepitas are great for those with lowered immunity, acne, poor wound healing and irregular ovulation.

PESTO – a great source of 'good' fats and nutrition, pesto is made from basil, olive oil, garlic, pine nuts and parmesan cheese. If you eat dairy-free, parmesan cheese can be replaced with cashews. Pesto is really easy to make at home by blending the above ingredients, although ready-made versions are common. When buying a ready-made product, check that olive oil has not been replaced with the cheaper and hormone-unfriendly canola oil or another vegetable oil. Pesto is versatile and is delicious in salads, stirred through vegetables or served with eggs for an extra boost of protein and 'good' fats, which really help to increase satiety from your meal.

PRUNES – also known as dried plums, prunes are a well-known digestive support. Prunes contain fibre in addition to sorbitol, a type of sugar that loosens the stool. Prunes have also been shown to increase the absorption of iron into the body. As with all dried fruits, prunes should be enjoyed in moderation and remember to only eat as many prunes as you would eat whole plums! For constipation, try making a chia gel with diluted prune juice (see page 46) and drink before bed.

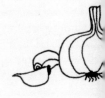

QUINOA – one of the few plant foods to be considered a complete protein. Quinoa contains good levels of magnesium, calcium, iron and phytonutrients. Quinoa is gluten-free and is known as a pseudograin. If you are avoiding grains, you are probably best to avoid quinoa as it does tend to irritate the gut and is often problematic in those with coeliac disease or inflammatory bowel disorders. I also recommend avoiding quinoa if you have an autoimmune disease. If you don't have any of these conditions and feel that you digest quinoa well, you can include it in moderation as either the whole seed (rinsed and soaked before cooking) or as the versatile quinoa flakes, often used as porridge or in baking. Quinoa is found in the health-food aisle of the supermarket, but you may need to venture to the health-food store to find quinoa flakes.

RAS EL HANOUT – this North African spice mix is used commonly in Moroccan cuisine and translates to 'head of the shop', meaning the best spices the shop has to offer. The blend includes cardamom, cloves, cinnamon, cumin, paprika and many more. These spices are warming, anti-inflammatory and great for hormonal health and longevity. Luckily for us, this tasty spice mix is inexpensive and readily available in the herb and spice section of most supermarkets. Ras el hanout is not a hot spice mix and is usually enjoyed by both children and adults.

RED CURRY PASTE – an antioxidant-rich blend of chilli, turmeric, garlic, lime and lemongrass. Check the ingredient list of ready-made pastes, as some may contain sugar, oils and artificial flavouring.

SALMON, SMOKED – a great source of protein and essential omega-3 fatty acids. Wild-caught salmon is better than farmed. Do your homework on the brand you buy, especially if it's something you consume on a regular basis. Your health is worth your time!

SALMON, TINNED – while fresh is always best, tinned salmon in moderation can provide you with an easy and inexpensive source of quality protein and calcium. To get the calcium, you need to make sure you are buying the tinned salmon with the bones, as it is the bones that provide the calcium, not the salmon itself. These bones are soft and work well in fish cakes or in an easy workday salad. If you're a tuna lover, try to rotate tuna with salmon to minimise mercury exposure. I recommend that tinned salmon only be consumed once a week; try to ensure you look for a sustainable brand that uses BPA-free packaging.

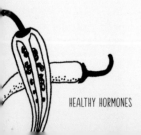

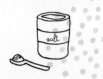

SALT – throw out the factory-produced table salt and invest in some nutrient-dense pink Himalayan rock salt. Pink Himalayan rock salt is a natural salt that can help to regulate water content in the body. If you are drinking lots of water, urinating frequently and still feeling thirsty, try adding a pinch of pink Himalayan rock salt to your water daily. The salt helps the body to absorb the water and most people will feel more hydrated, with less of those pesky bathroom trips!

SESAME OIL – contains high levels of natural antioxidants and has antibacterial and antiviral properties. Sesame oil is best used in moderation and should only be consumed cold, not heated. It gives a delicious nutty flavour to our Asian-style dressing (see page 200).

SESAME SEEDS – a great source of calcium, zinc, protein and good fats, sesame seeds have been used in food for more than 5000 years. They have a mild taste and are easy to sprinkle over salads, vegetables and meats for a nutrient boost. Sesame seeds are also used to make tahini, which is also incredibly nutritious and a great source of calcium and 'good' fats. The type of 'good' fats in sesame seeds are quite stable and less prone to rancidity than most other seeds. Look out for white or black sesame seeds in your local supermarket.

SUNFLOWER SEEDS – provide lots of vitamin E, selenium and magnesium in addition to protein and good fats. Sunflower seeds are great for hormonal balance and fertility as these nutrients, in combination with the 'good' fats, can help to promote healthy oestrogen levels and egg health for optimal fertility and pre-conception support. Look for untoasted seeds that are not loaded with artificial flavourings, ideally organic if possible. Sunflower butter, similar to peanut butter or almond butter, is a great way to consume sunflower seeds and makes a tasty snack with apple or celery for kids who usually can't take nut products to school. Sunflower butter is available at health-food stores and some supermarkets.

TAHINI – a paste made from sesame seeds, tahini is a great source of protein, calcium and 'good' fats. Tahini is found in the health-food aisle of most supermarkets and is available as hulled or unhulled. Unhulled tahini is full of nutrients and is one of the richest sources of calcium available. Tahini (hulled) is lighter in colour, more processed and stripped of some nutrients, although it still contains the good-quality protein and 'good' fats. Hulled tahini has a milder flavour and can be used to balance the stonger taste of unhulled tahini in dressings if needed. Unhulled tahini is a key ingredient in hummus and is also delicious drizzled over steamed vegetables, used as a dip or added to porridges, smoothies and baked goods.

TAMARI – this gluten-free version of soy sauce is made from fermented soy beans and doesn't contribute to the potentially unwanted hormonal effects of other soy products. Tamari is great as a dipping sauce or for use in Asian-inspired recipes, dressings and stir-fries. A great cupboard staple.

TOMATO PASTE (concentrated purée) – this Mediterranean staple is a convenient way to use tomatoes in cooking. High in vitamin C, vitamin K and potassium, tomato paste is relatively unprocessed and should contain tomatoes as its only ingredient. Tomato paste is also a rich source of antioxidants, in particular lycopene, which may help to reduce the risk of certain cancers. Tomato paste is inexpensive and widely available at supermarkets. Make sure you choose a product packaged in glass as opposed to plastic tubs, tubes or foil sachets, which may contain hormone-damaging chemicals.

TURMERIC – a powerful anti-inflammatory and antioxidant spice, I use high-dose supplemental turmeric in my clinic to support liver health, reduce inflammation and pain of conditions such as endometriosis, uterine fibroids, period pain, headaches, backache, joint pain and digestive dysfunction. Turmeric can be used daily in food; add it to smoothies or try a Turmeric chai (see page 231). I always sprinkle turmeric onto scrambled eggs for an easy morning boost. For the conditions listed above, it may be best to also consider a turmeric supplement for optimal dose and results.

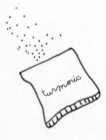

VANILLA BEAN – has a delicious taste and has been used for centuries to improve mood and mental performance. Vanilla bean powder or paste can be added to smoothies and baked goods to give them a sweet taste without the need for added sugar. Avoid vanilla essence and look for pure vanilla paste or dried vanilla beans. Whole vanilla beans can be expensive, but some supermarkets now stock vanilla bean pieces in a grinder, similar to a salt grinder, which is more affordable and lasts for longer! Look for this product in the baking section of the supermarket and use vanilla liberally in smoothies, porridges, chia puddings, baked goods and on yoghurt for that sweet vanilla taste.

YOGHURT – many people are confused as to which yoghurt is the most nutritious. Most of the yoghurts in the supermarket are what I would affectionately call 'dairy desserts', full of sugar and lacking the probiotic benefits of real yoghurt. Ideally look for a full-fat, organic yoghurt that does not contain any added sugar, fillers or flavours. The ingredient list should only contain whole milk and live cultures. Sheep or goat's yoghurt are also options for those who don't tolerate cow's milk or who would like to increase the nutrient variety in their diets. For those who are dairy-free, avoid soy yoghurt and look for an unsweetened coconut yoghurt, which should only contain coconut milk and live cultures.

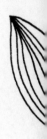

ZOODLES – made from zucchini (courgettes), zoodles are made with a special kitchen appliance called a spiraliser, which is widely available and relatively cheap. Zoodles can be eaten raw or lightly steamed, depending on your preference for the texture. Zoodles look just like spaghetti so they are a great substitute for pasta and can be used as a base for salads, or just stir some pesto through for a simple side dish.

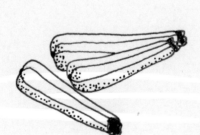

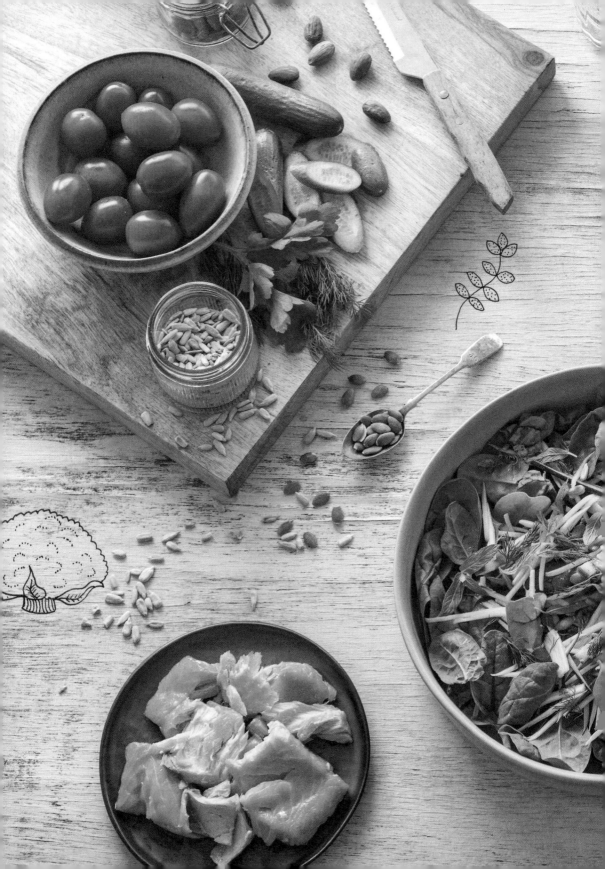

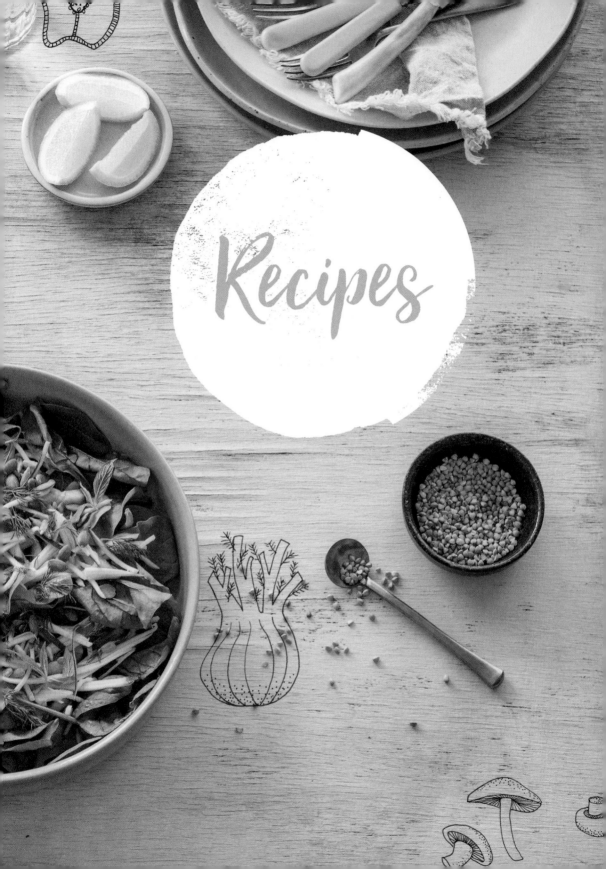

Recipes

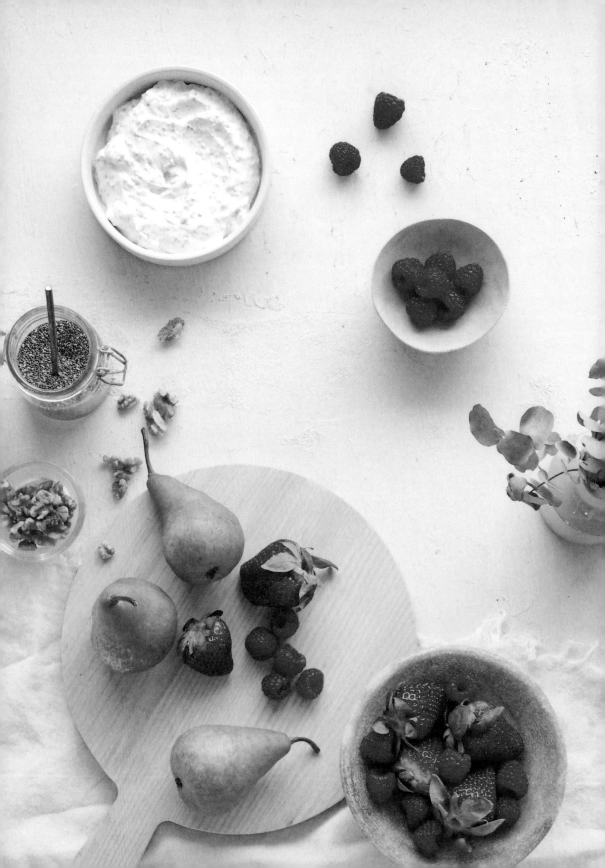

Breakfast

·····································

Yoghurt pots

These are hands-down the easiest breakfast food to make in advance and set yourself up for the week ahead. They contain the perfect blend of protein, 'good' fats and something fresh and can also be made into a snack size for between meals. Look for a natural yoghurt that does not contain any added sugar in the ingredient list. If you are used to sweet yoghurts, try preparing these in advance and top with frozen raspberries or fresh passionfruit, which will blend through and sweeten the yoghurt. If your diet is dairy free, try them with a coconut yoghurt.

PREPARATION 5 MINS
MAKES 1 POT

200 g (7 oz/¾ cup) plain or Greek-style yoghurt
1 tablespoon chia seeds
1 teaspoon vanilla paste
1 tablespoon LSA (linseed, sunflower seed and almond) meal

Stir together all of the ingredients and leave in the fridge for at least 15 minutes.

OPTIONS

★ Just before serving, add a handful of raspberries and three or four brazil nuts, coarsely chopped.

★ Slice a peach, roughly chop five or six toasted almonds and add a tablespoon of toasted pepitas (pumpkin seeds).

★ Stir in 1 tablespoon of shredded coconut and top with sliced banana, five or six chopped cashews and the grated zest of half a lime.

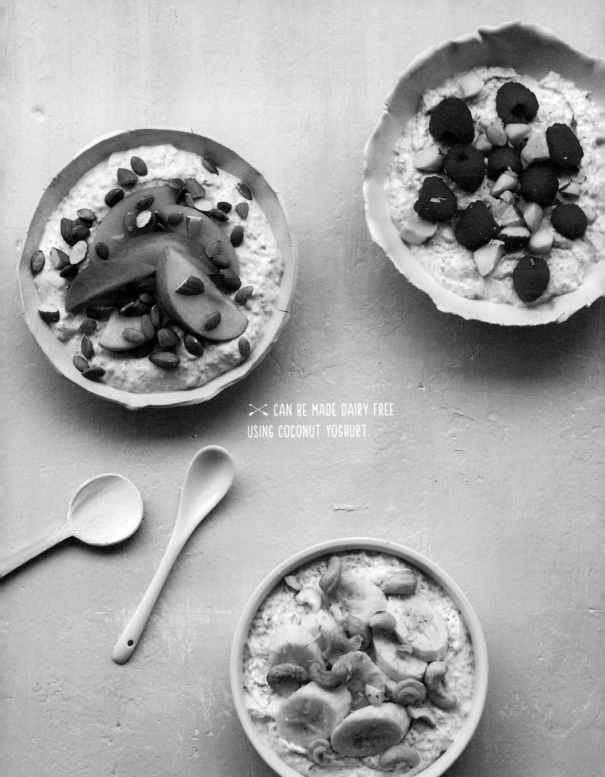

CAN BE MADE DAIRY FREE
USING COCONUT YOGHURT.

Scrambled eggs
WITH BROCCOLI & CAULIFLOWER

Eating seven types of veggies a day is easy when you start with this yummy dish. Who knew broccoli and cauliflower could taste great in the morning? These veggies aren't the first thing you think of for breakfast but they work well, helping to move excess oestrogen out of your body, which makes this recipe great for those suffering from PMS, period pain and endometriosis or who are trying to conceive.

PREPARATION 5 MINS
COOKING 20 MINS
SERVES 2

6–8 cherry tomatoes
1 teaspoon olive oil, plus 1 tablespoon extra
1 brown onion, thinly sliced
150 g (5½ oz) cauliflower, thinly sliced
100 g (3½ oz) broccoli, thinly sliced
4 eggs, whisked
15 g (½ oz/¼ cup) chopped flat-leaf (Italian) parsley
35 g (1¼ oz/¼ cup) crumbled feta cheese
micro herbs, for serving

Turn the oven to 200°C (400°F). Put the cherry tomatoes in an ovenproof dish, drizzle with 1 teaspoon of olive oil and season with salt and pepper. Put the tomatoes straight into the oven while it's heating up: this will ensure the tomatoes are ready in time.

Heat the remaining olive oil in a medium non-stick frying pan, add the onion and fry, stirring, for 2 minutes.

Add the cauliflower and broccoli and cook, stirring, for a further 8–10 minutes, until lightly golden.

Pour on the whisked eggs and season with salt and pepper. Stir gently for a few minutes, then continue cooking until eggs are almost cooked through. Add the parsley and finish cooking.

To serve, scatter the feta and micro herbs on top and serve with the roasted cherry tomatoes.

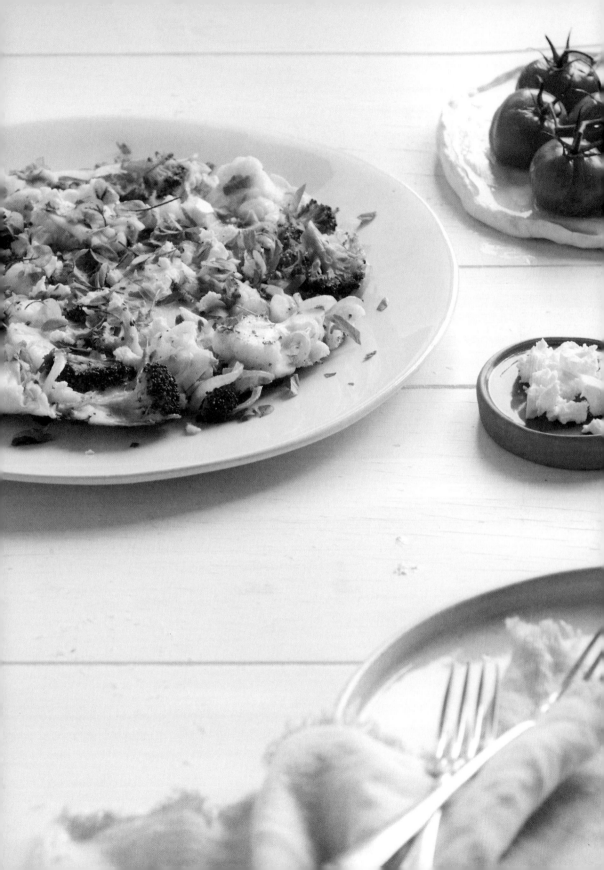

Red chilli lentils AND haloumi

This weekend breakfast is a great way to start the day with a nutrient-dense vegetarian meal filled with protein, iron and fibre. Try batch-cooking the lentil mixture and keeping the leftovers in the freezer ready for another meal.

PREPARATION 15 MINS
COOKING 20 MINS
SERVES 2

205 g (7¼ oz/1 cup) red lentils
1 tablespoon olive oil
1 small onion, chopped
2 garlic cloves, chopped
2 tablespoons tomato paste (concentrated purée)
½ fresh red chilli, finely chopped
2 eggs
4 slices of haloumi
baby spinach leaves, to serve

Rinse the red lentils under cold water and discard any brown bits. Heat the olive oil in a medium frying pan and add the onion. Cook for a few minutes, then add the garlic and cook for a few more minutes to soften. Add the red lentils, 500 ml (17 fl oz/2 cups) of water, the tomato paste and chilli; season with pepper and stir to combine.

Bring to the boil, then reduce to a simmer and cook for 10–12 minutes, stirring occasionally.

While the lentils are cooking, cook the eggs to your liking (soft- or hard-boiled) and heat a small frying pan over medium heat. Fry the haloumi slices for approximately 2 minutes each side until lightly golden on both sides.

To serve, divide the cooked lentils between two serving bowls and top each one with two slices of haloumi and a peeled egg. Add a good handful of spinach leaves. Season with salt.

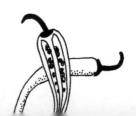

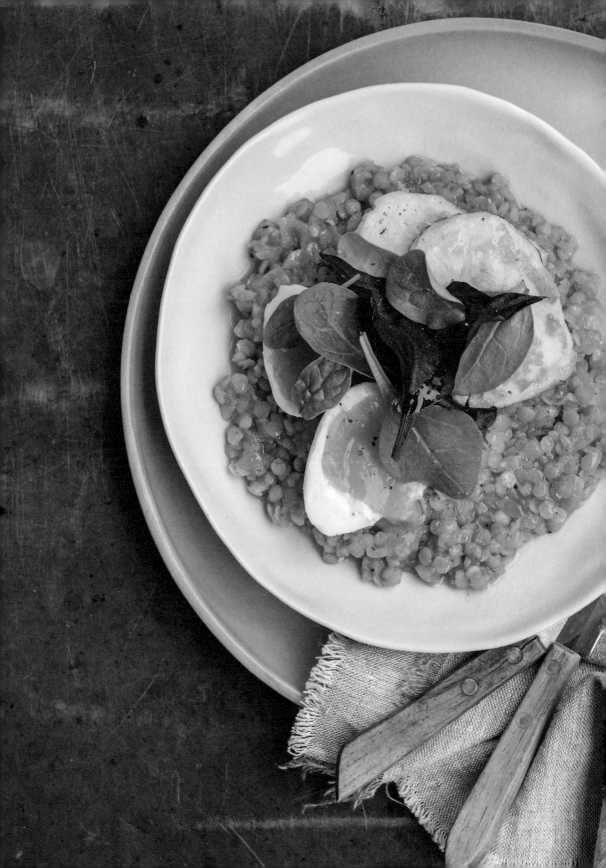

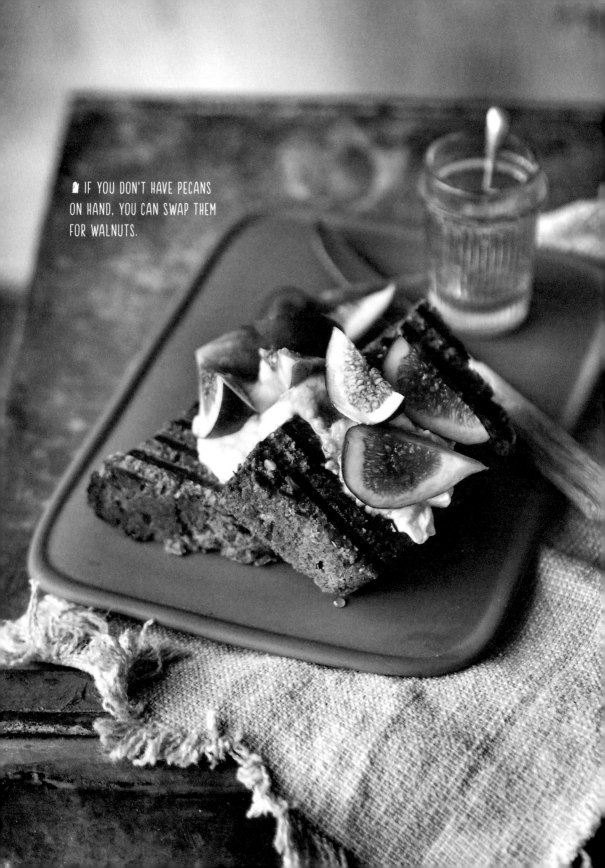

IF YOU DON'T HAVE PECANS ON HAND, YOU CAN SWAP THEM FOR WALNUTS.

Nutty banana bread

Having some grain-free, nutrient-dense snacks on hand means that making good food choices is a breeze. I make this banana bread all the time for my family, who are always looking for a snack. It's great for using up ripe bananas and I often make a double batch and put one in the freezer. It also doubles as an easy breakfast that ticks all the boxes! Try it toasted in a sandwich press for the ultimate treat, enjoy a slice as a snack and spread with some good-quality nut butter.

PREPARATION 15 MINS
COOKING 50 MINS

3 ripe bananas
4 eggs
2 tablespoons coconut oil
100 g (3½ oz/1 cup) almond meal
30 g (1 oz/¼ cup) coconut flour
60 g (2¼ oz/½ cup) coarsely chopped pecans
45 g (1½ oz/½ cup) desiccated coconut
45 g (1½ oz/¼ cup) dried apricots, sliced
40 g (1½ oz/¼ cup) sliced dates
40 g (1½ oz/¼ cup) sunflower seeds
40 g (1½ oz/¼ cup) linseeds (flaxseeds)
1 teaspoon baking powder
2 teaspoons ground cinnamon, plus extra (optional)
1 apple, thinly sliced (optional)

Preheat the oven to 180°C (350°F). Grease and line an 11 x 22 cm (4¼ x 8½ inch) baking tin.

In a large bowl, mash the bananas, add the eggs and coconut oil and mix well. In a separate large bowl, combine all of the other ingredients, except the apple and extra cinnamon, and stir. Add the contents of one bowl to the other and stir until combined.

Pour the batter into the prepared baking tin and lay the apple slices on top with an extra sprinkle of cinnamon (if using).

Bake for 50 minutes or until a skewer inserted into the centre comes out clean.

Serve the bread toasted with ricotta and fruit.

Mushroom AND ricotta crêpes

Despite its name, buckwheat is a seed and does not contain any wheat or gluten.
It is full of protein, magnesium and B vitamins. In keeping with our philosophy of
prepping as much as possible in advance, these crepes can be frozen and reheated.
Try making a double batch and using them to make toasted crêpe wraps for lunch.
For best freezing results, lay a sheet of baking paper between each one.

PREPARATION 15 MINS
COOKING 15 MINS
SERVES 2

1 tablespoon olive oil
1 French shallot, finely chopped
1 tablespoon butter
300 g (10½ oz) brown mushrooms, quartered
1 teaspoon coriander seeds
1 teaspoon sage leaves, finely chopped
1 teaspoon rosemary leaves, finely chopped
1 handful rocket (arugula) leaves
1 tablespoon chopped walnuts
3 teaspoons ricotta cheese

CRÊPES

100 g (3½ oz/¾ cup) buckwheat flour
2 eggs
250 ml (9 fl oz/1 cup) milk
butter, for frying

★ THESE VERSATILE
CREPES CAN BE SERVED
FOR BREAKFAST, LUNCH
OR DINNER.

Put the olive oil and shallot in a medium frying pan and cook over
medium heat for a few minutes. Add the butter, mushrooms, coriander
seeds, sage and rosemary and cook gently for about 10 minutes, then
add a few tablespoons of water to get the pan juices flowing.

While this is cooking, make the crêpes. Combine the ingredients in
a bowl and whisk together. Melt some butter in a medium frying pan.
Pour in a small amount of batter and spread evenly to cover the pan as
thinly as possible. Cook until you see bubbles form, then flip the crêpe
over. They take a few minutes each side. Repeat to make a second crêpe.

To serve, place a crêpe on each plate and divide the mushroom mixture
between them on one half of each crêpe. Top with some rocket, walnuts
and ricotta, then fold the crêpe over and serve.

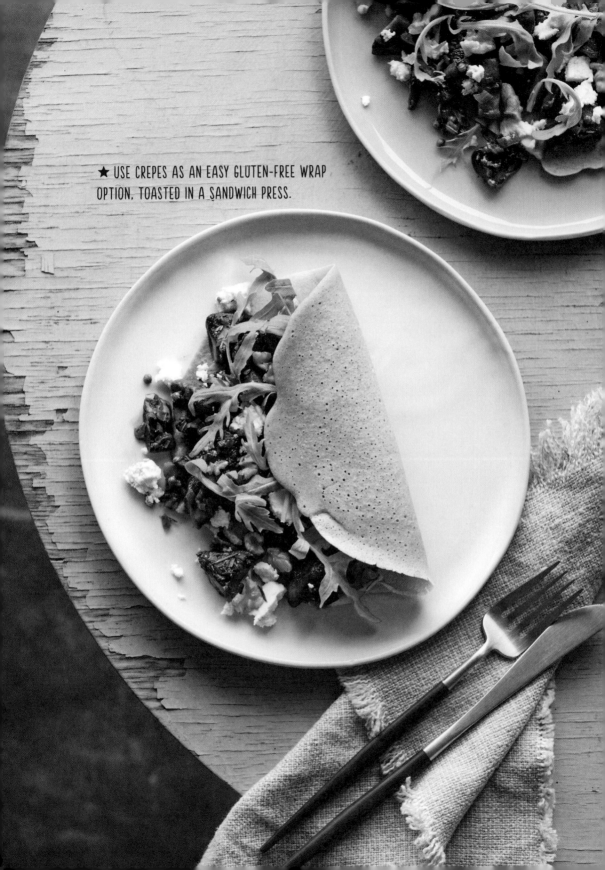

★ USE CREPES AS AN EASY GLUTEN-FREE WRAP OPTION, TOASTED IN A SANDWICH PRESS.

Egg stack

This tasty combination of eggs served with hormone-friendly avocado is given extra flavour with the tang of pesto, chilli and lemon. The protein in the eggs and the 'good' fats in the avocado should help stabilise blood-sugar levels and leave you feeling satisfied. This is a perfect breakfast for people with PCOS or those trying to crowd out excess grains from their diet. Eggs can be hard-boiled in advance to make this an easy workday breakfast. If you eat breakfast at work, simply pop it into a container the night before and add the avocado just before eating.

PREPARATION 10 MINS

COOKING 5 MINS

SERVES 1

½ avocado
juice of ¼ lemon
1 large handful of baby spinach leaves
2 eggs, soft-boiled, hard-boiled or poached
¼ fresh red chilli, thinly sliced
1 tablespoon Kale & mint pesto (see page 169)

Prepare the eggs as you like them. Mash the avocado with a fork and mix in the lemon juice. Place a big handful of spinach leaves on a plate and top with the eggs. Add the mashed avocado and serve with the fresh chilli and pesto.

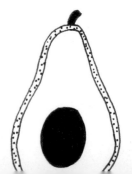

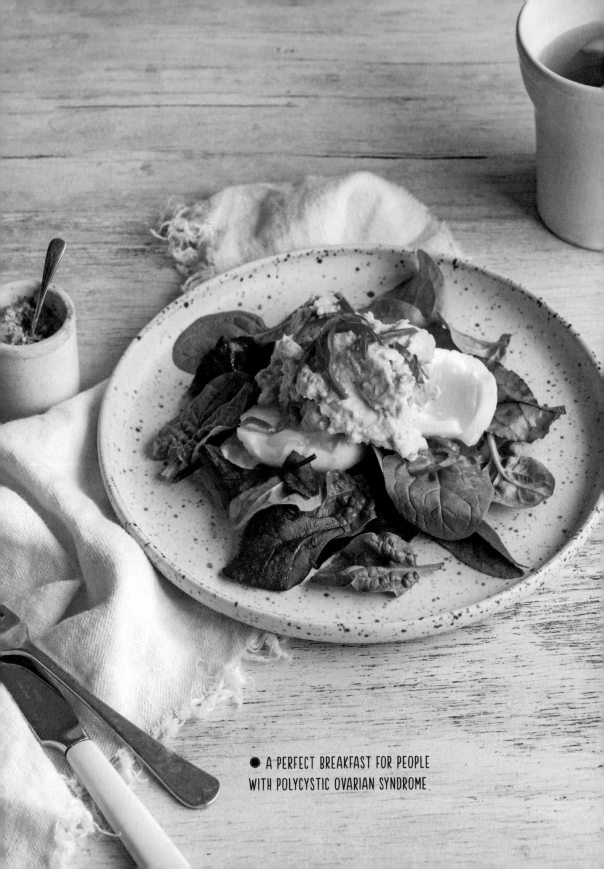

A PERFECT BREAKFAST FOR PEOPLE
WITH POLYCYSTIC OVARIAN SYNDROME.

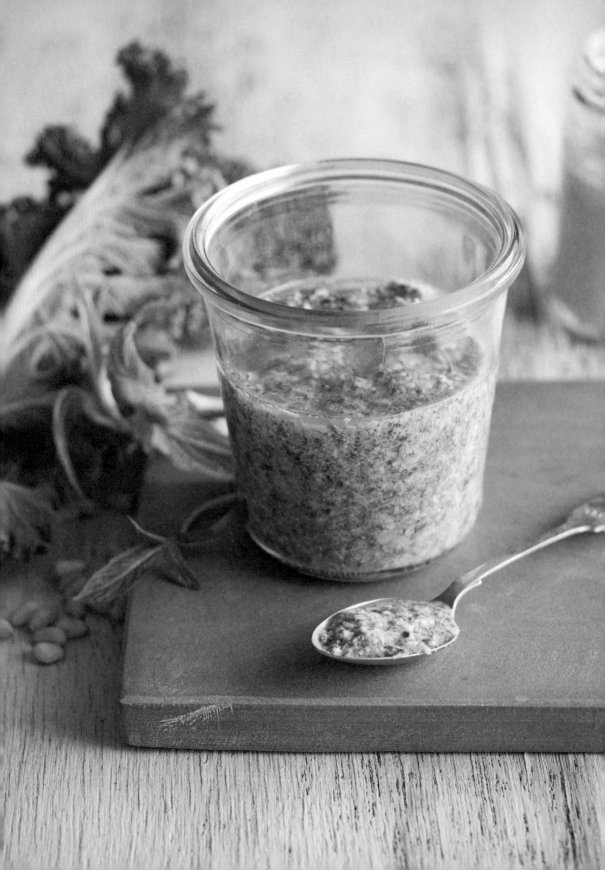

Kale and mint pesto

Pesto is one of those wonderful condiments that goes with so many things and adds lots of extra nutrients and flavour. It's very easy to make, so try different combinations of herbs, leaves and nuts to find your favourite taste.

PREPARATION 5 MINS
MAKES 250 G (9 OZ/1 CUP)

2 kale leaves, stems removed
1 handful of mint leaves
1½ teaspoons capers
1 teaspoon dijon mustard
1 garlic clove
40 g (1½ oz/¼ cup) pine nuts
60 ml (2 fl oz/¼ cup) extra virgin olive oil
grated zest and juice of 1 lemon

Combine all of the ingredients in a deep bowl and season with salt and pepper. Using a handheld blender, blend all the ingredients until you have a slightly chunky paste. Store in a container in the fridge and add to anything!

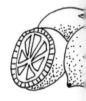

Chia porridge

When I first discovered chia porridge, I was surprised at how a recipe without oats could be so warming and satisfying. Chia is a great source of omega-3, which makes it the perfect choice for a hormone-balancing breakfast. This recipe is also useful for reducing inflammation and improving oestrogen levels, making it a perfect choice for those with endometriosis. Once you are familiar with the recipe it is easy to change the flavours: for example, replace the banana with grated apple and cinnamon. This is definitely a winter staple.

PREPARATION 5 MINS
COOKING 5 MINS
SERVES 2

40 g (1½ oz/¼ cup) chia seeds
60 ml (2 fl oz/¼ cup) milk (you can use almond or coconut),
    plus extra to serve
½ banana, mashed
1 teaspoon vanilla paste
2 tablespoons LSA (linseed, sunflower seed and almond) meal

TOPPINGS

1 tablespoon toasted hazelnuts, coarsely chopped
1 tablespoon raspberries
1 teaspoon pomegranate seeds
1 teaspoon currants

Place all ingredients in a saucepan with 185 ml (6 fl oz/¾ cup) of water and stir continuously over low heat for about 5 minutes.

To serve, add the toppings and a drizzle of milk. You can also serve with yoghurt and Fruit compote (see page 172).

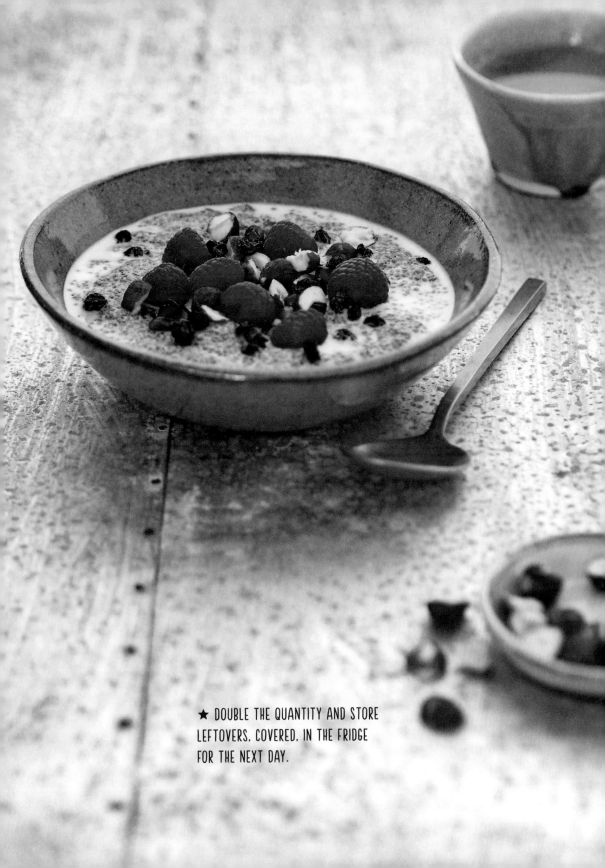

★ DOUBLE THE QUANTITY AND STORE
LEFTOVERS, COVERED, IN THE FRIDGE
FOR THE NEXT DAY.

Fruit compote

This compote is easy to make in bulk and freeze in batches. You can then add it to chia puddings and yoghurt pots as a quick and easy sweetener.

PREPARATION 5 MINS
COOKING 20 MINS

4 apples, peeled and cut into wedges
5–6 plums, cut into wedges
1 teaspoon ground cinnamon (or 1 cinnamon stick)
1 teaspoon ground allspice
1 teaspoon vanilla paste (or 1 vanilla bean, halved lengthways)
3 star anise

Put all of the ingredients into a large saucepan and cover with water. Stir and bring to the boil. Reduce to a simmer and cook, stirring occasionally, for 15–20 minutes until the fruit is soft and the water has reduced slightly. Allow to cool, then store the compote in an airtight container in the fridge for 1 week or in portions in the freezer for up to 3 months.

◖ IF PLUMS ARE OUT OF SEASON, USE PEARS AND HALF A CUP OF PITTED PRUNES.

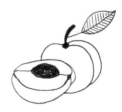

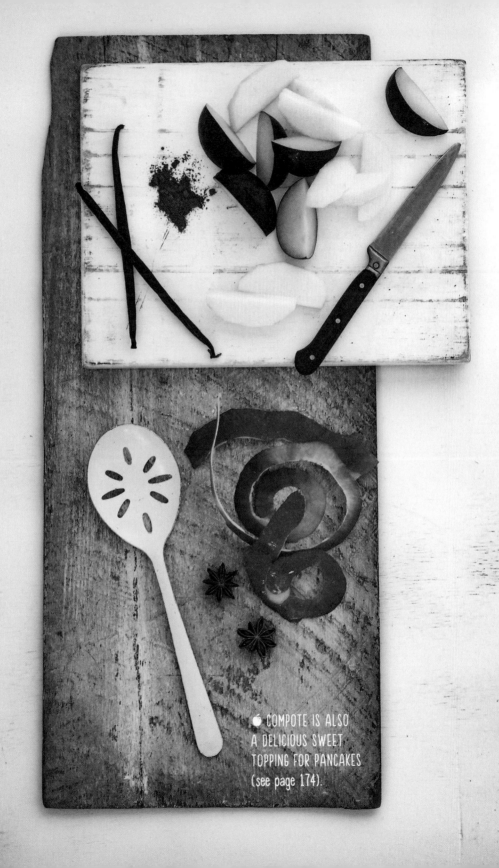

COMPOTE IS ALSO
A DELICIOUS SWEET
TOPPING FOR PANCAKES
(see page 174).

Banana pancakes
WITH BERRIES

These pancakes are sweet, delicious and super easy to prepare. They are grain-free, high in protein and perfect for those who like to start the day with something sweet. Try them after dinner for a quick dessert (my whole family loves them). Almond meal is an easy way to bump up the hormone-friendly 'good' fats in your breakfast: these are a little slower to cook than flour-based pancakes, but are well worth the wait.

PREPARATION 5 MINS
COOKING 15 MINS
SERVES 1–2 (3 PANCAKES)

1 banana
2 eggs
1 teaspoon ground cinnamon
1 teaspoon vanilla paste
25 g (1 oz/¼ cup) almond meal
½ apple, grated
butter, for frying
yoghurt, blueberries and raspberries, to serve

Using a handheld blender or food processor, combine all of the ingredients (except the apple) and blend well. Add the grated apple.

Heat a large frying pan over low to medium heat, melt the butter and pour in a third of the pancake mix. Cook until small bubbles appear (about 2 minutes), then gently flip and cook for a further 1–2 minutes on the other side. Repeat with the remaining batter. The best way to cook these is slowly and for longer than flour-based pancakes.

Serve with yoghurt and seasonal fresh berries.

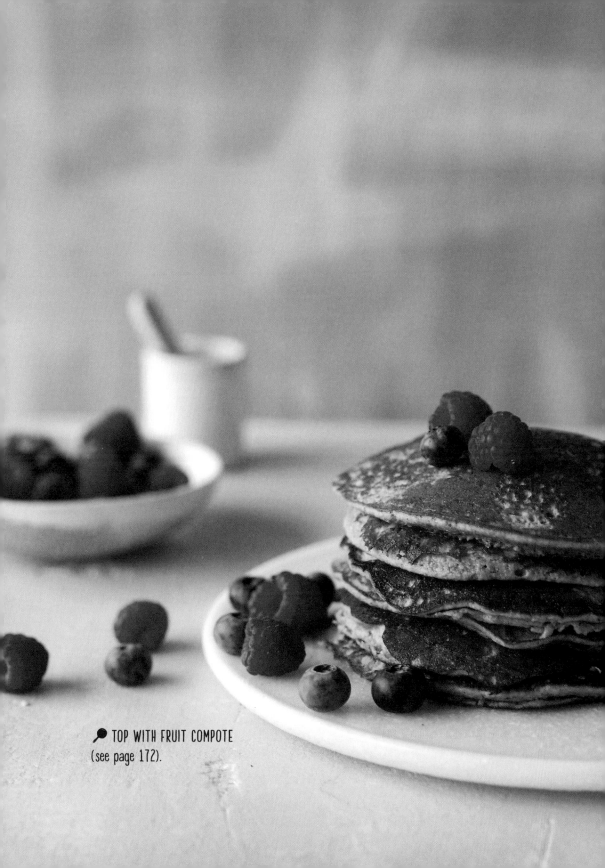

TOP WITH FRUIT COMPOTE
(see page 172).

Fruit and seed slice

The ingredients in this slice are rich in vitamin B6 and magnesium, which are essential for progesterone production and may help to regulate menstruation, boost mood and reduce PMS. The dried figs, nuts and seeds are also rich sources of calcium and should be included regularly in the diet for optimal bone health and to support oestrogen production.

PREPARATION 10 MINS
MAKES 16 BARS

150 g (5½ oz/1 cup) brazil nuts
160 g (5¾ oz/1 cup) almonds
160 g (5¾ oz/1 cup) pitted dates
7 dried figs
40 g (1½ oz/¼ cup) chia seeds
grated zest of 1 orange
juice of ½ orange
75 g (2¾ oz/½ cup) sunflower seeds
75 g (2¾ oz/½ cup) pepitas (pumpkin seeds)
1 tablespoon finely chopped rosemary

Combine all of the ingredients in a food processor and blitz until they start to come together as a batter. You may need to add a little more orange juice, 1 tablespoon at a time.

Spread onto a baking tray lined with baking paper and press out evenly. Smooth over with a spatula so that it's nice and flat.

Leave in the fridge for at least 1 hour or overnight. Lift off the tray and cut into 16 snack-size pieces. Store in an airtight container in the freezer for up to 3 months.

✎ WHILE YOU HAVE THE FOOD PROCESSOR OUT, MAKE UP SOME BLISS BALLS (see page 204) SO THAT YOU ARE STOCKED UP ON NUTRITIOUS SNACKS.

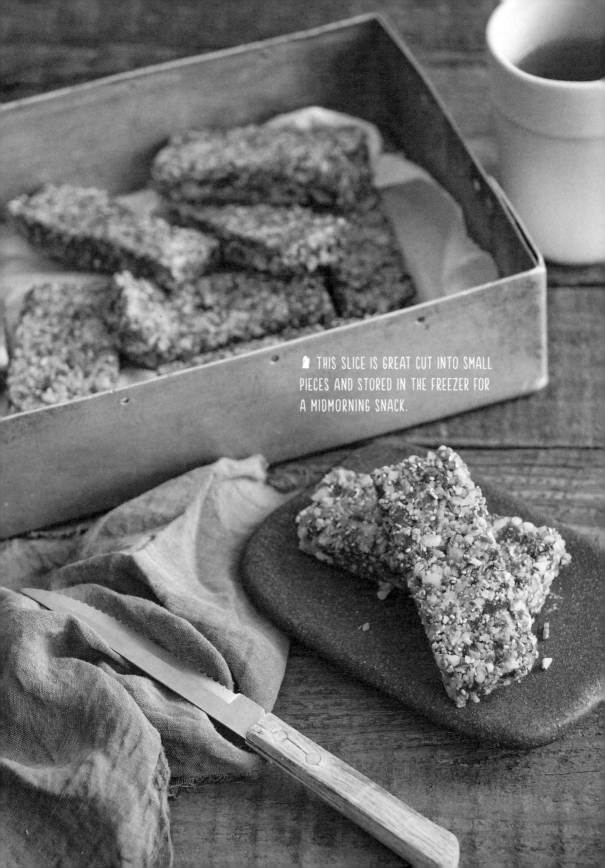

THIS SLICE IS GREAT CUT INTO SMALL PIECES AND STORED IN THE FREEZER FOR A MIDMORNING SNACK.

Smoothies

These are great choices for hormone health. Blend all of the ingredients thoroughly, until smooth (you might need to shake the blender halfway through).

PREPARATION 5 MINS
SERVES 1

WINTER SMOOTHIE

20 g (¾ oz/1 handful) rocket (arugula) or baby spinach
2 tablespoons walnuts
¾ small ripe pear, cored and chopped
1 tablespoon chopped fresh ginger
1 orange, peeled and chopped
50 g (1¾ oz) ice

SUMMER SMOOTHIE

150 g (5½ oz) pineapple pieces
½ lemon, peeled and chopped
1 small handful of mint leaves
2 small kale leaves, stems removed, or 1 small handful baby spinach leaves
1 teaspoon chia seeds
75 ml (2¼ fl oz) water
50 g (1¾ oz) ice

CHOCOLATE TREAT SMOOTHIE

30 g (1 oz) cashews
1½ teaspoons raw cacao powder
2 pitted dates (ideally soaked in boiled water in advance) or ½ frozen banana
150 ml (5 fl oz) almond milk
150 g (5½ oz) ice

BERRY RIPE

1 teaspoon raw cacao powder
1 banana
60 g (2¼ oz) frozen raspberries
100 ml (3½ fl oz) coconut milk
50 g (1¾ oz) ice

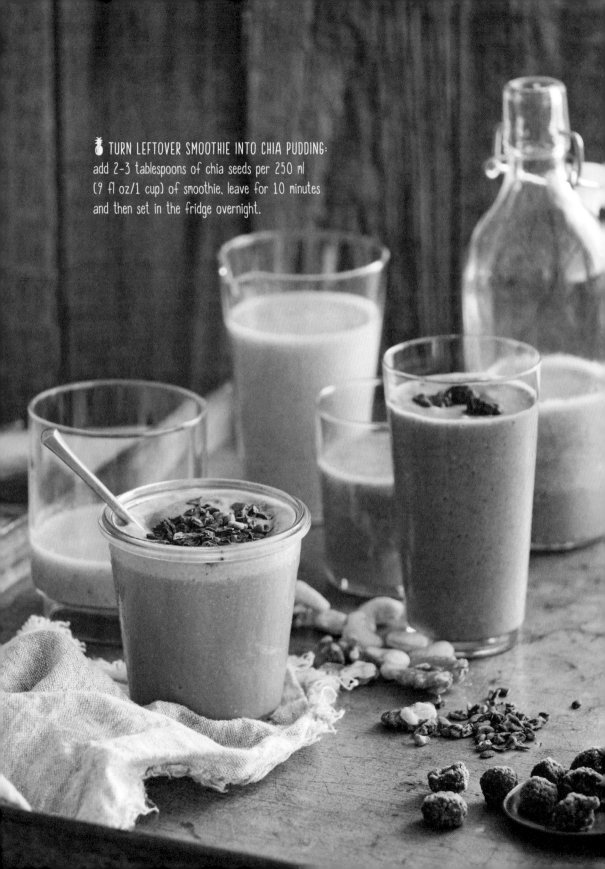

🍍 TURN LEFTOVER SMOOTHIE INTO CHIA PUDDING:
add 2-3 tablespoons of chia seeds per 250 ml
(9 fl oz/1 cup) of smoothie, leave for 10 minutes
and then set in the fridge overnight.

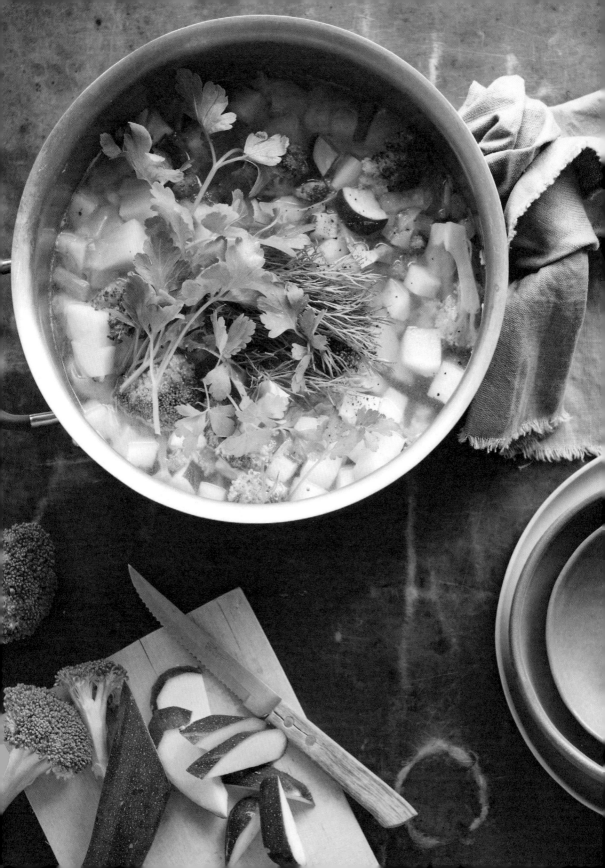

Lunch

··

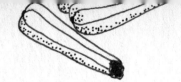

Toasties

Use the buckwheat crêpes recipe (or defrost previously made crêpes from the freezer) and add fillings before toasting in a sandwich press for a perfect healthy lunch.

PREPARATION 5 MINS
COOKING 30 MINS
MAKES 7 CREPES

BUCKWHEAT CRÊPES

135 g (4¾ oz/1 cup) buckwheat flour
250 ml (9 fl oz/1 cup) milk
2 eggs
butter, for frying

Combine the ingredients in a bowl and whisk them together. Melt some butter in a medium frying pan and pour in a small amount of the batter, spreading it evenly to cover the base of the pan as thinly as possible. Cook until you see bubbles form, then flip over. The pancakes take a few minutes on each side.

Heat an electric sandwich press. Make up the toasties on a separate board and then cook in the press until crispy on the outside.

FILLINGS

★ Poached chicken, pesto and rocket (arugula)

★ Zucchini (courgette) ribbons, sundried tomato, feta cheese, basil and pine nuts

★ Tuna, baby capsicum (pepper), tomato and bocconcini

★ Sliced banana, peanut butter and shredded coconut

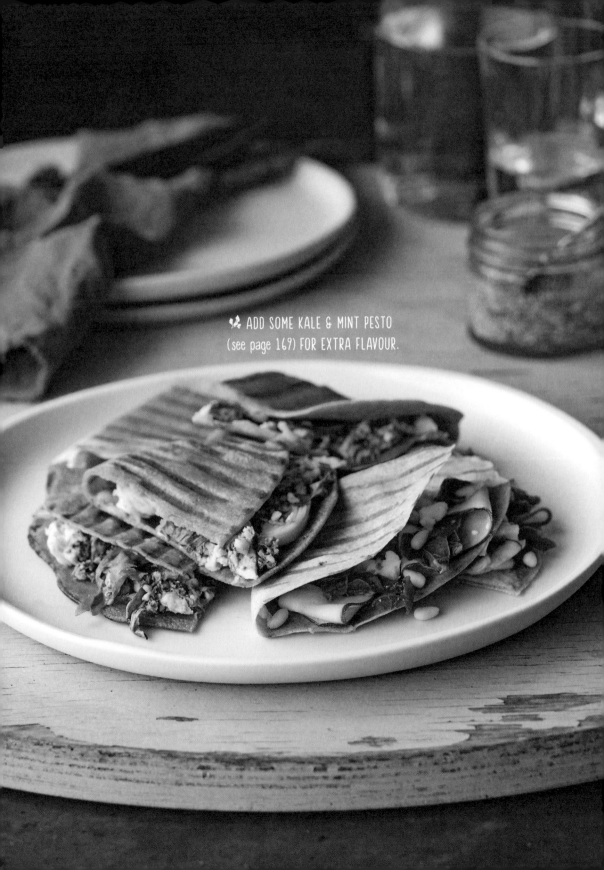

ADD SOME KALE & MINT PESTO
(see page 169) FOR EXTRA FLAVOUR.

Seed crackers

Sometimes you just need something crunchy to eat! These crackers are great to have on hand for an easy satisfying lunch, or to serve with soup. The linseeds (flaxseeds) are excellent for those with PCOS as they help to keep blood-sugar levels stable with their unique combination of fibre, 'good' fats and protein. Don't worry if a few crumbs break off, just use them to scatter onto other food. Keep any leftover toasted seeds in a container ready to put on salads and soups.

PREPARATION 10 MINS
COOKING 50 MINS
MAKES 10 CRACKERS

160 g (5¾ oz/1 cup) linseeds (flaxseeds)
⅓ cup mixed sunflower seeds, pepitas (pumpkin seeds), chia seeds
   and sesame seeds
3 tablespoons almond meal
2 teaspoons garlic powder
1 teaspoon smoked paprika
olive oil spray, for greasing

Preheat the oven to 180°C (350°F). Line a baking tray with baking paper. Combine all the ingredients in a bowl with 310 ml (10¾ fl oz/1¼ cups) of water and stir. Set aside for 15 minutes.

🍶 IF YOU HAVE ANY MIXTURE LEFT OVER, SPREAD IT OVER A SECOND TRAY AND THEN BREAK UP AFTER BAKING TO MAKE DIPPING CRACKERS.

Spray the baking tray with olive oil spray and press the mixture evenly onto the tray to about 5 mm (¼ inch) thick. Use a knife to cut the mixture into 10 rectangles; that way they will be easy to cut when they are cooked.

Bake for 30 minutes. Take the tray out of the oven and cut along the lines again. Return to the oven and bake for a further 20 minutes.

Cool the crackers on the tray, then break along the lines and store in an airtight container for 1 month.

TOPPING IDEAS

These crackers are great to take with you for a nutritious and delicious lunch. Enjoy them with any of the dips on page 188.

avocado dressing (page 194), mango, chopped macadamias, jalapeños, sashimi-grade tuna, coriander (cilantro) • smoked salmon, avocado, walnuts, feta cheese, lemon • coconut chicken (page 211), cucumber, cashews, mint • hummus, cherry tomatoes, black olives, dukkah

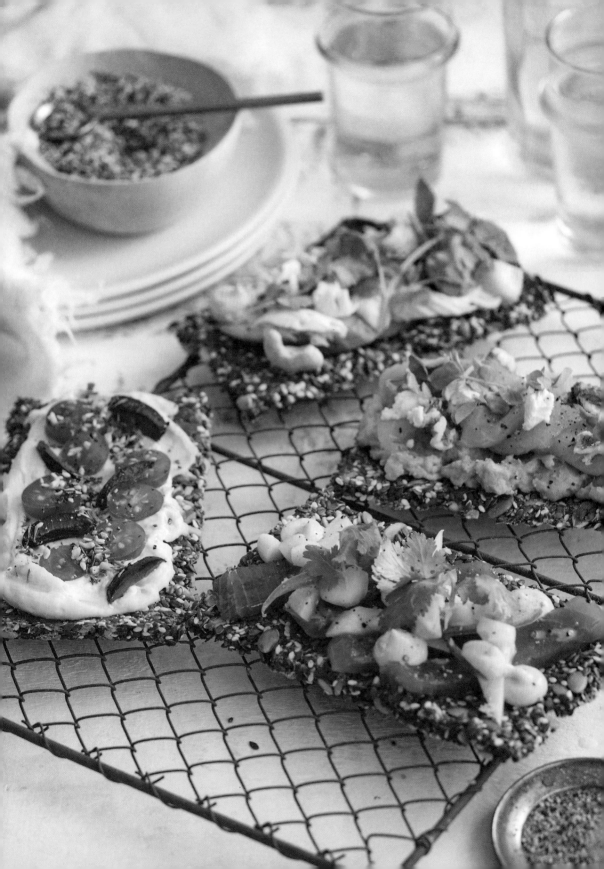

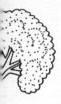

Super green soup

This nutritious soup is quick and easy to make and features great ingredients for detoxing and cleansing. The addition of garlic, leek and onion also means that this soup has the immune-boosting benefits of being antibacterial and antiviral. As with most soups, it will taste better the next day when all the flavours have had time to mingle together. Make extra and freeze in smaller batches.

PREPARATION 20 MINS
COOKING 35 MINS
SERVES 4

1 tablespoon extra virgin olive oil
2 leeks, chopped
1 onion, chopped
3 garlic cloves, coarsely chopped
1 bunch asparagus, coarsely chopped
1 small broccoli, coarsely chopped
2 zucchini (courgettes), coarsely chopped
1 large potato, chopped
2 handfuls of herbs (parsley and mint are great)
1 litre (35 fl oz/4 cups) organic chicken broth
280 g (10 oz/2 cups) frozen baby peas
1 handful baby spinach leaves, plus 5–6 extra to serve
1 tablespoon ricotta cheese, to serve
5 toasted almonds, coarsely chopped, to serve

Heat the olive oil in a heavy-based frying pan, add the leek, onion and garlic and cook for a few minutes until softened. Season with salt and pepper.

Add all of the ingredients except the peas and spinach. Cover with water to 3 cm (1¼ inches) above the top of the vegetables. Bring to the boil, then reduce to a simmer and cook for about 30 minutes. Add the peas and spinach and cook for a further 2 minutes. Purée until very smooth.

To serve, top with the creamy ricotta, spinach leaves and roasted almonds.

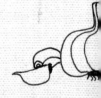

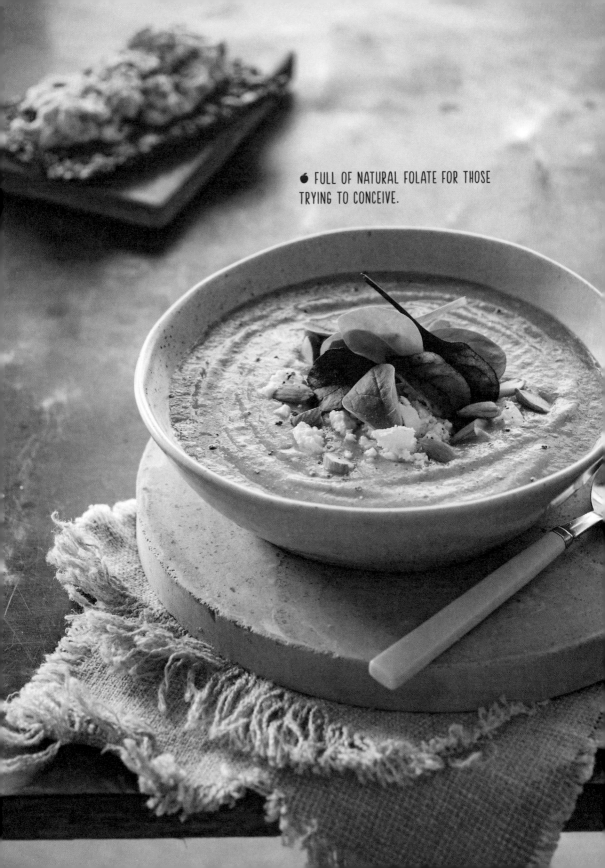

FULL OF NATURAL FOLATE FOR THOSE TRYING TO CONCEIVE.

Dips

Serve these with raw vegetables or spread on Seed crackers (page 184) as a light lunch.

Serve these with raw vegetables or spread on Seed crackers (page 184) as a light lunch.

PREPARATION 10 MINS
MAKES ABOUT 350 G
(12 OZ/1½ CUPS)

SUPER GUACAMOLE

1½ avocados
1 tablespoon lime juice
⅓ capsicum (pepper), chopped
1 handful of coriander (cilantro)
5–6 cherry tomatoes, chopped

2 teaspoons sunflower seeds
1 tablespoon cooked corn
  kernels (off the cob)
finely chopped chilli or
  jalapeño, optional

Mash the avocado and mix with all the remaining ingredients.

PREPARATION 15 MINS
MAKES ABOUT 500 G
(1 LB 2 OZ/2 CUPS)

THAI SWEET POTATO DIP

1 sweet potato, chopped
3 teaspoons red curry paste
80 g (2¾ oz/½ cup) cashews
2 tablespoons coconut milk
1 teaspoon tamari
3 tablespoons olive oil

1 handful of coriander (cilantro),
  plus extra leaves for topping
juice of ½ lime
1 teaspoon ground turmeric
chilli and chopped cashews or
  toasted coconut, for topping

Boil the sweet potato in water for 10 minutes or until soft. Drain and mix in a food processor (or with a handheld blender) with the remaining ingredients. Add water, a tablespoon at a time, until the dip has a smooth consistency. Top with coriander, chilli, cashews or coconut.

PREPARATION 5 MINS
MAKES ABOUT 340 G
(11¾ OZ/1½ CUPS)

WHITE BEAN + GARLIC DIP

400 g (14 oz) tin butter beans or
  cannellini beans, drained
1 small garlic clove
grated zest and juice of 1 lemon
2 tablespoons tahini
2 tablespoons olive oil

1 teaspoon ground sumac
1 teaspoon ground cumin
1 teaspoon paprika
olive oil, toasted pine nuts
  and pomegranate seeds,
  for topping

Combine all of the ingredients in a food processor, season with salt and pepper and blitz until smooth. Add water if needed, a tablespoon at a time, until the dip has a smooth consistency. Top with a drizzle of olive oil, toasted pine nuts and pomegranate seeds.

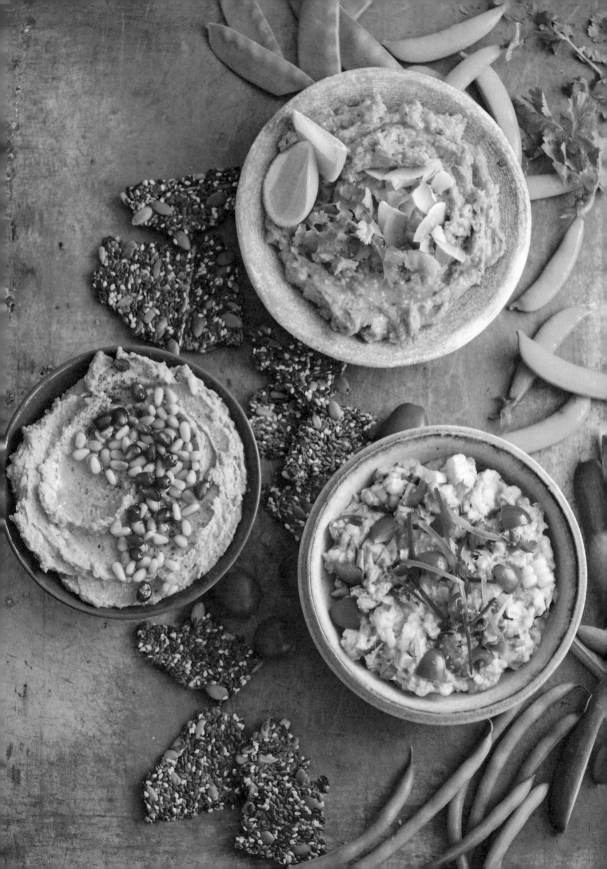

Roasted cauliflower soup

The cauliflower in this hearty soup makes it really creamy and even people who don't love cauliflower will probably enjoy this dish. Cauliflower is a member of the brassica family of vegetables, known for their hormone-balancing and oestrogen-clearing effects. If you use fresh chicken bone broth, you will also get the extra digestive health and nutritional benefits. The feta, parsley and hazelnut toppings really make this dish special, but you could also use the Creamy tahini dressing (see page 200).

PREPARATION 20 MINS
COOKING 1 HOUR 20 MINS
SERVES 4

1 whole cauliflower
2 large onions or 4 small ones, cut into wedges
1 fennel bulb, cut into wedges
6 garlic cloves
olive oil spray
1 potato, chopped
2 tablespoons thyme leaves
2 teaspoons ground cardamom
2 teaspoons ground cumin
1 teaspoon paprika
1 litre (35 fl oz/4 cups) chicken bone broth or stock
milk (optional)
parsley, feta cheese and roasted hazelnuts, for topping

Preheat the oven to 200°C (400°F). Line 2 large baking trays with baking paper.

Chop cauliflower into small chunks, about 4 cm (1½ inches). Spread the cauliflower chunks, onion and fennel wedges and whole garlic cloves on the prepared trays and season with salt and pepper.

Spray with olive oil and roast for 40 minutes or until vegetables are lightly golden.

Put the roasted vegetables in a large saucepan, removing the soft roasted garlic from the skin. Add the potato, thyme, cardamom, cumin, paprika and the chicken broth. You may have to add a little extra water to cover the vegetables.

Bring to the boil, then reduce the heat and simmer for about 30 minutes. Blitz with a handheld blender until very smooth. Add a little milk for a creamier soup. Serve with chopped parsley, crumbled feta and chopped hazelnuts.

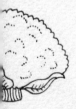

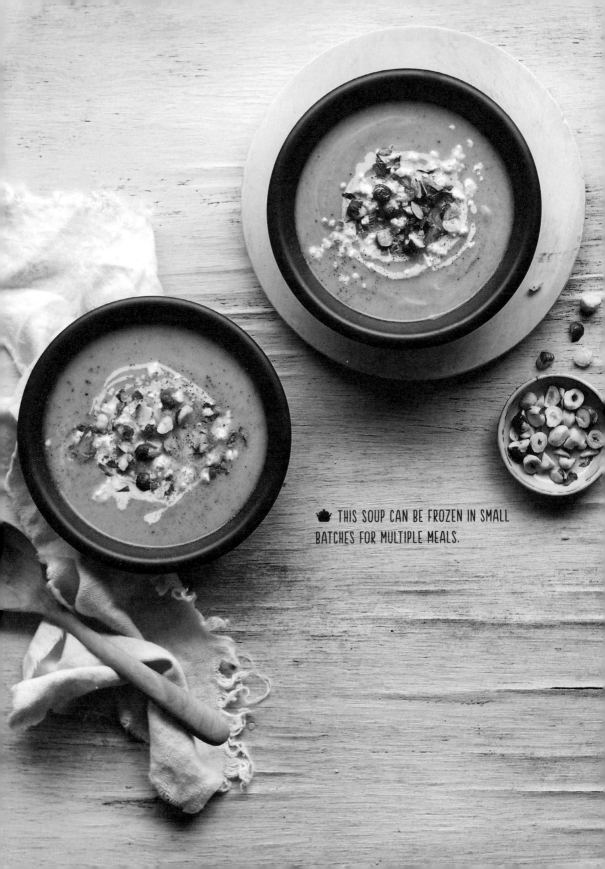

THIS SOUP CAN BE FROZEN IN SMALL BATCHES FOR MULTIPLE MEALS.

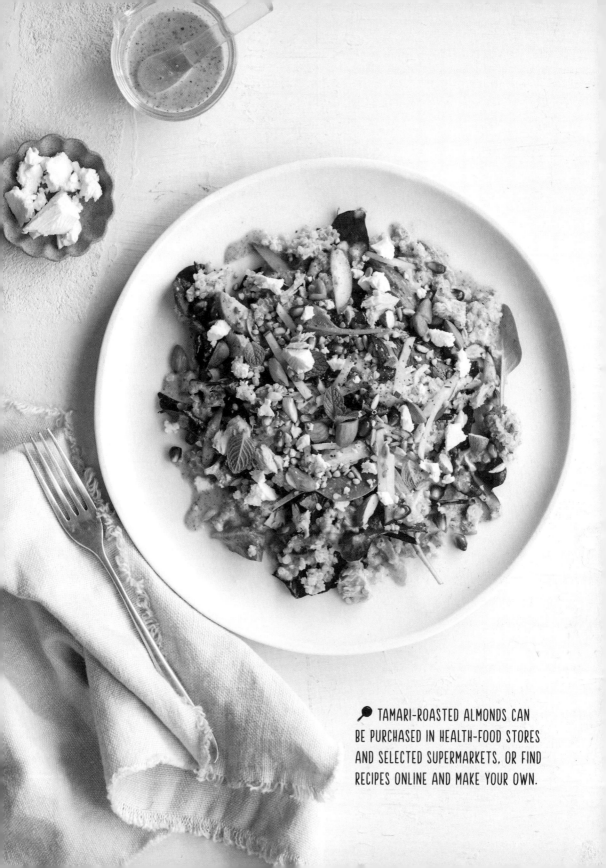

TAMARI-ROASTED ALMONDS CAN BE PURCHASED IN HEALTH-FOOD STORES AND SELECTED SUPERMARKETS, OR FIND RECIPES ONLINE AND MAKE YOUR OWN.

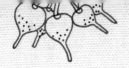

Quinoa salad with tuna

This simple salad can be easily doubled for more lunches or a light dinner. Cook extra quinoa to use in another lunch or for making the yummy Quinoa-crusted chicken (see page 222) for dinner. Buckwheat groats are fantastic seeds that are not only nutritious but really crunchy. Just put them in a medium frying pan and stir for a few minutes until lightly golden and crisp.

PREPARATION 10 MINS
SERVES 1-2

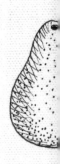

½ cup cooked quinoa
1 handful of spinach leaves
95 g (3¼ oz) tin tuna
¼ Lebanese (short) cucumber, sliced
¼ avocado, sliced
1 radish, sliced into matchsticks
1 teaspoon buckwheat groats, toasted
1 teaspoon sunflower seeds
1 tablespoon pomegranate seeds
1 tablespoon crumbled feta cheese
1 tablespoon tamari-roasted almonds
herbs, such as parsley and dill, for topping
Green herb dressing (see page 200)

Combine the quinoa, spinach, tuna, cucumber, avocado and radish in a bowl. Top with buckwheat groats, sunflower seeds, pomegranate seeds, feta, almonds and herbs. Dress with Green herb dressing and season with salt and pepper.

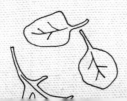

Coleslaw with chicken
AND AVOCADO DRESSING

This coleslaw is a must for anyone with symptoms of relative oestrogen excess such as fluid retention, weight gain, moodiness, endometriosis or subfertility. The cabbage and radish in this recipe both contain a compound known as diindoylmethane (DIM), which helps to remove excess oestrogen through the liver and has also been studied for its effectiveness in combating breast cancer.

PREPARATION 30 MINS
COOKING 15 MINS
SERVES 2

MAYO
PREPARATION 20 MINS
MAKES 225 G (8 OZ/1 CUP)

500 g (1 lb 2 oz) chicken breast
270 ml (9½ fl oz) coconut cream
2 cups finely shredded wombok (Chinese cabbage)
75 g (2¾ oz/1 cup) finely shredded red cabbage
140 g (5 oz/1 cup) finely shredded fennel
15 g (½ oz/¼ cup) chopped dill
15 g (½ oz/¼ cup) chopped flat-leaf (Italian) parsley
2 radishes, julienned
1 tablespoon toasted sunflower seeds

1 tablespoon toasted buckwheat groats
1 tablespoon toasted pepitas (pumpkin seeds)

AVOCADO DRESSING

40 g (1½ oz/¼ cup) cashews
½ avocado
2 tablespoons lemon juice
1 tablespoon olive oil
1 tablespoon tahini
1 tablespoon caramelised red wine vinegar

Put the chicken breast in a saucepan and add the coconut cream. Top up with water so the chicken is completely covered with liquid. Bring to the boil, then reduce to a simmer and cook for 12–15 minutes until the chicken is cooked through. Leave the chicken to rest in the liquid for 5 minutes, then remove and thinly slice or shred with a fork.

In a separate bowl, combine both types of cabbage with the fennel, dill and parsley. Toss to combine and divide between two bowls. Top with the shredded chicken, radish, sunflower seeds, buckwheat groats and pepitas and season with salt and pepper.

To make the avocado dressing, place the cashews in a bowl, cover with hot water and soak for 15 minutes. Meanwhile, put the avocado, lemon juice, olive oil, tahini and red wine vinegar in a smoothie maker or food processor. Season with salt and pepper and add 80 ml (2½ fl oz/⅓ cup) of water. After the cashews have cooled, drain and add to the rest of the ingredients and blitz until very smooth. Drizzle a generous amount of the avocado dressing over the salad.

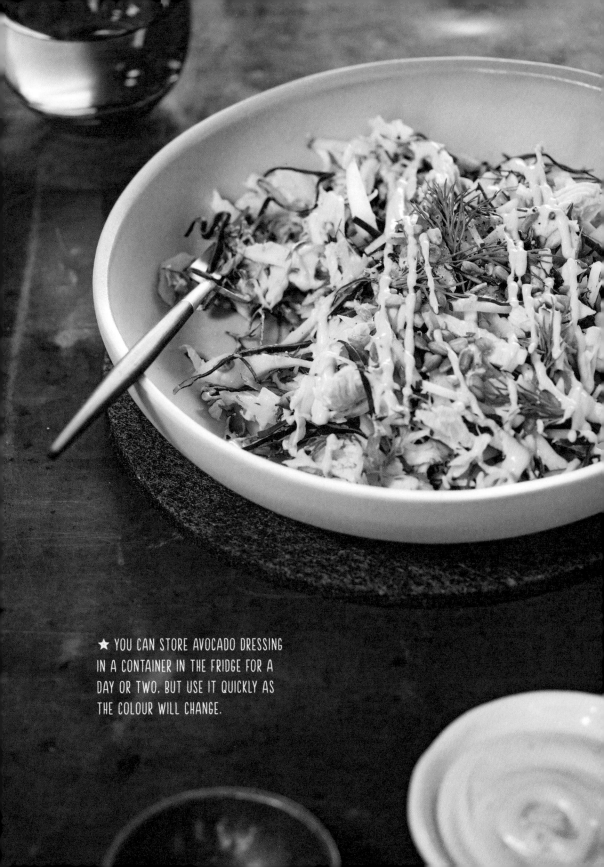

★ YOU CAN STORE AVOCADO DRESSING IN A CONTAINER IN THE FRIDGE FOR A DAY OR TWO. BUT USE IT QUICKLY AS THE COLOUR WILL CHANGE.

Kale AND broccoli salad

This super green salad goes well with most meals but is also really good on its own. Simply add some leftover chicken, tuna or salmon for a nutritious lunch. This salad may help relieve relative oestrogen excess, so add it to your regular diet if you suffer from fatigue, easy weight gain, sugar cravings, heavy periods or mood swings. If you are making this recipe for just yourself, you'll have enough for at least two lunches, so add the avocado and dressing just before serving. This salad is best when chopped quite finely, like a tabouleh salad.

PREPARATION 15 MINS
SERVES 2-3

1 small broccoli (just the very tops)
1 kale leaf, stem removed and finely sliced
½ Lebanese (short) cucumber, chopped
15 g (½ oz/½ cup) chopped flat-leaf (Italian) parsley
8 cherry tomatoes, quartered
3 tablespoons pomegranate seeds
1 tablespoon sunflower seeds
1 tablespoon chopped tamari-roasted almonds
1 tablespoon pepitas (pumpkin seeds)
1 tablespoon currants
1 avocado, chopped
squeeze of lemon juice
Green herb dressing (see page 200), for topping

Combine all of the ingredients in a bowl and mix together. Season with salt and pepper and top with plenty of the Green herb dressing.

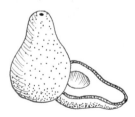

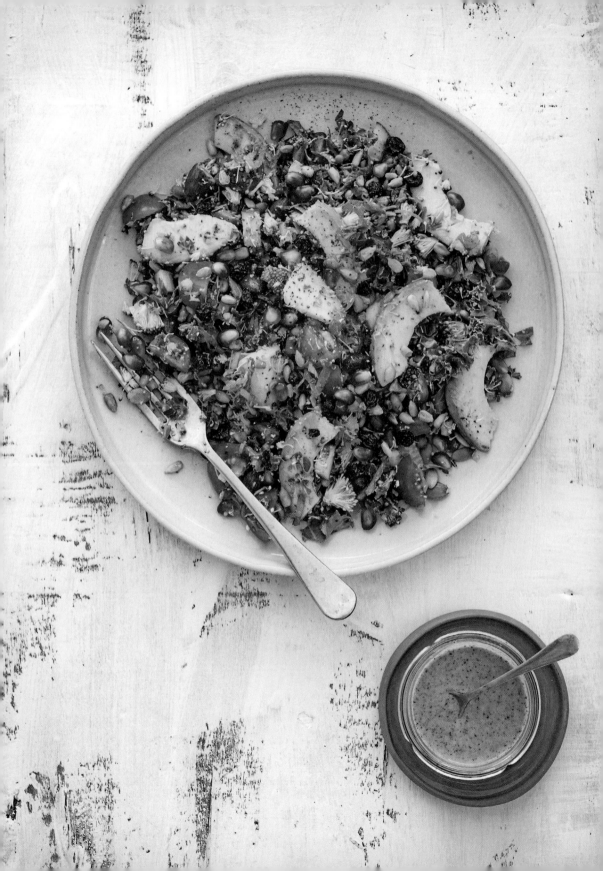

Big frittata

With so much focus on protein, it can be a nice change to have a vegetarian
meal that still contains protein (thanks to the eggs and cheese). The mushrooms
in this recipe are a source of selenium, which helps to support optimal fertility
and a healthy thyroid. This recipe is particularly recommended for those with
autoimmune thyroid issues. This is a perfect dish to slice and freeze and use
for lunches or a quick dinner. Serve with a simple salad.

PREPARATION 10 MINS
COOKING 1 HOUR 5 MINS
SERVES 8

1 sweet potato, chopped
olive oil, for roasting and frying
1 brown onion, thinly sliced
200 g (7 oz) Swiss brown mushrooms (about 10), coarsely chopped
12 eggs
185 g (6 fl oz/¾ cup) milk
50 g (1¾ oz/½ cup) grated cheddar cheese (or cheese of your choice)
1 zucchini (courgette), grated
45 g (1½ oz/1 cup) baby spinach leaves
1 tablespoon thyme leaves
100 g (3½ oz) cherry tomatoes, halved
60 g (2¼ oz) goat's cheese

Preheat the oven to 200°C (400°F). Line a baking tray with baking paper.

Spread the sweet potato on the tray, spray with olive oil and season with
salt and pepper. Roast for about 15 minutes. Meanwhile, cook the onion
and mushrooms in a medium frying pan with 1 tablespoon of oil for
about 10 minutes until soft.

Line a large baking dish with baking paper and spray with oil. Turn the
oven down to 180°C (350°F).

Whisk the eggs in a bowl and add milk, grated cheese and grated
zucchini. Stir until combined.

Spread the onion, mushrooms, baby spinach leaves and roasted sweet
potatoes in the prepared baking dish and pour the egg mixture over. Top
with thyme leaves, cherry tomatoes and crumble the goat's cheese over.
Bake for about 50 minutes until the egg has set.

Slice and serve with a salad and a good-quality tomato chutney.

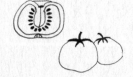

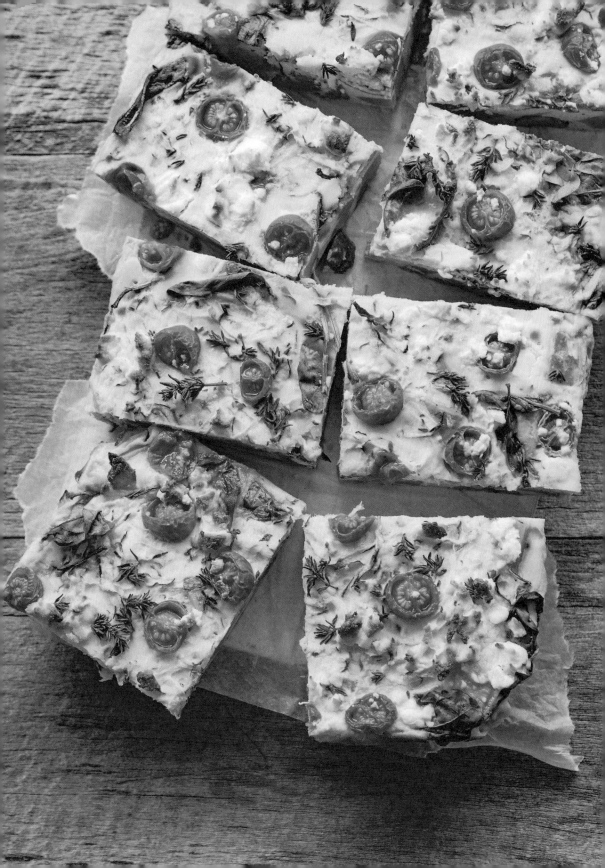

Dressings

Dressings are important for bringing a dish together and adding an extra punch of flavour as well as a boost of nutrients. Making your own dressings means that you can use quality, fresh ingredients that are nutritious and hormone-friendly. These tasty dressings and sauces not only give a zesty flavour to your food but they also contain important antioxidants and anti-inflammatory ingredients.

PREPARATION 5 MINS
MAKES 200 G (7 OZ/1 CUP)

CREAMY TAHINI DRESSING

2 tablespoons hulled tahini
2 tablespoons hummus
3 tablespoons plain yoghurt

1 teaspoon ground cumin
grated zest and juice of
½ orange

Put all of the ingredients in an airtight container, stirring well as you add each ingredient. Season with salt and pepper. Store in the fridge for up to 1 week. Serve with meat, fish and roasted veggies (I'd eat it with anything).

PREPARATION 5 MINS
MAKES ABOUT 130 G
(4½ OZ/1 CUP)

GREEN HERB DRESSING

2 tablespoons olive oil
2 tablespoons macadamia oil
2 teaspoons caramelised red
    wine vinegar
2 teaspoons water

1 large handful of mint
1 large handful of flat-leaf
    (Italian) parsley
1 small garlic clove
juice of ½ lemon

Put all of the ingredients in your smoothie maker or blender, season with salt and pepper and blitz until smooth. If you do not use it all at once, it can be stored in the fridge but its green colour will not stay as bright.

PREPARATION 5 MINS
MAKES ABOUT 125 ML
(4½ FL OZ/½ CUP)

ASIAN-STYLE DRESSING

1 tablespoon macadamia oil
1 tablespoon rice wine vinegar
1 tablespoon sesame oil
1 tablespoon tamari or soy sauce
1 teaspoon fish sauce (or to taste)

2 teaspoons honey
juice of ½ lime
1 kaffir lime leaf
1 heaped teaspoon grated
    fresh ginger

Put all of the ingredients in a container with a tight-fitting lid and shake it up to mix together. Leave the kaffir lime leaf in the container. Store in the fridge for up to 1 month.

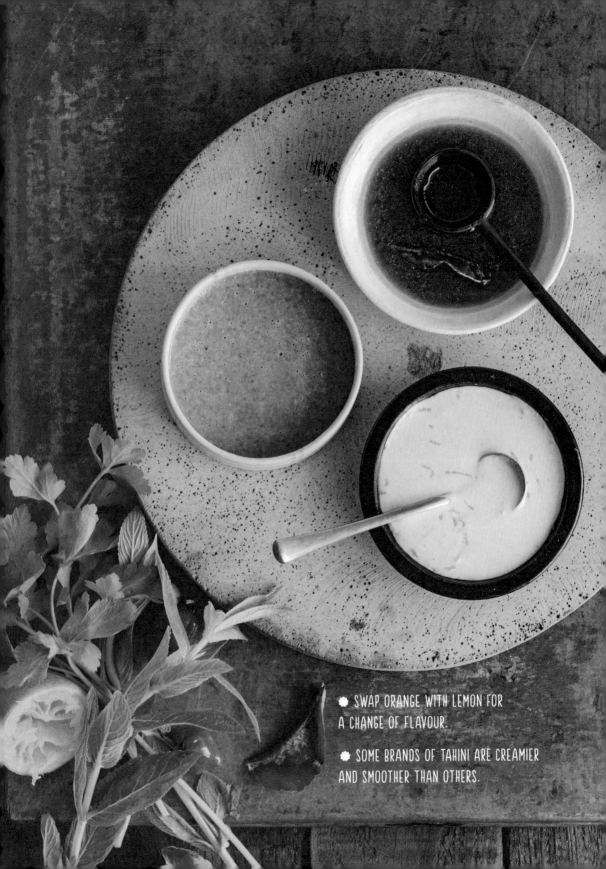

❀ SWAP ORANGE WITH LEMON FOR
A CHANGE OF FLAVOUR.

❀ SOME BRANDS OF TAHINI ARE CREAMIER
AND SMOOTHER THAN OTHERS.

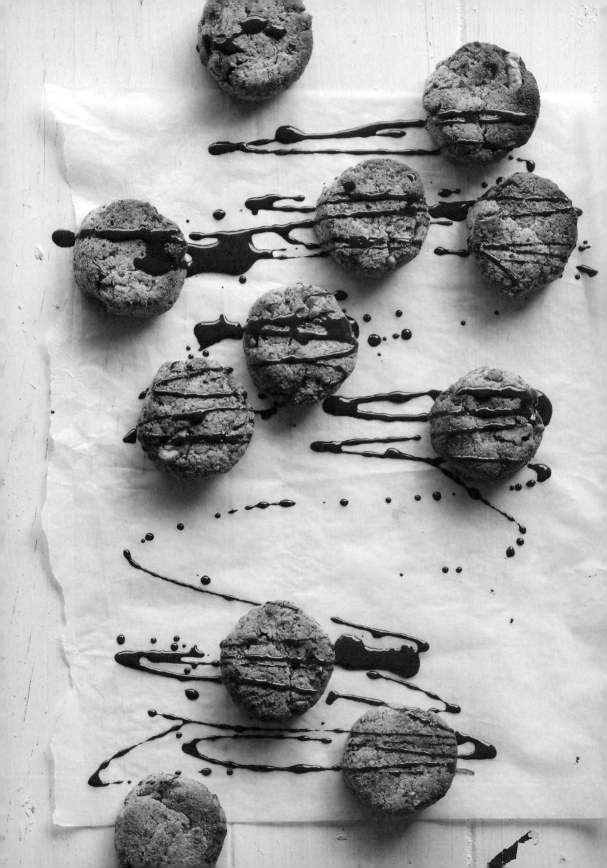

Nut biscuits

These biscuits are a great treat to take into the office so that you are not tempted by the office biscuit tin after lunch! They are full of nutritious ingredients and are a great source of protein and 'good' fats, essential for boosting concentration and focus. These biscuits are also a great source of fibre, which is important for a healthy digestive system and supporting hormonal balance.

PREPARATION 10 MINS
COOKING 20 MINS
MAKES 12 BISCUITS

100 g (3½ oz/1 cup) almond meal
30 g (1 oz/¼ cup) coconut flour
2 tablespoons desiccated coconut
30 g (1 oz/¼ cup) chopped walnuts
40 g (1½ oz/¼ cup) chopped dates
80 g (2¾ oz) butter, melted
1 teaspoon vanilla paste
1 tablespoon pear juice concentrate
1 tablespoon honey
1 egg, whisked
chocolate drizzle (optional): 1 teaspoon raw cacao powder
    mixed with 1 teaspoon coconut oil

Preheat the oven to 180°C (350°F). Line a baking tray with baking paper.

Put the almond meal, coconut flour, desiccated coconut, walnuts and dates in a bowl and mix well.

In a separate small bowl, stir together the butter with the vanilla, pear juice concentrate and honey. Add to the almond mixture. Add the egg and mix well so that it all comes together like dough.

Roll small amounts of the mixture into flattened balls and place them on the tray, leaving a space between each ball. Bake for 20 minutes or until slightly golden on the edges.

For the chocolate drizzle, melt the ingredients in the microwave for about 1 minute and drizzle over the top of the biscuits.

🍐 PEAR JUICE CONCENTRATE CAN BE BOUGHT IN HEALTH-FOOD STORES.

Bliss balls

Bliss balls are the perfect afternoon snack to satisfy sweet cravings and keep your energy levels high. For each recipe below, put all the ingredients except the water and topping in a food processor and blitz together. Gradually add the water until the mixture just comes together (test by pinching a small amount between your fingers). Roll tablespoons of the mixture into balls, scatter the topping on a tray and roll the balls in it. Store in an airtight container in the freezer for up to 3 months. They defrost quickly, so are easy to eat on the go!

PREPARATION 10 MINS

EACH RECIPE MAKES 12 BALLS

APRICOT + COCONUT BLISS BALLS

85 g (3 oz/½ cup) pitted dates
55 g (2 oz/¼ cup) pitted prunes
    (about 8)
8 dried apricot halves
45 g (1½ oz/½ cup) desiccated
    coconut

80 g (2¾ oz/½ cup) cashews
1 teaspoon chia seeds
1 tablespoon pepitas (pumpkin
    seeds)
1 teaspoon ground cinnamon
1 tablespoon water

PEANUT BUTTER + CHOCOLATE BLISS BALLS

110 g (3¾ oz/½ cup) pitted
    prunes
40 g (1½ oz/¼ cup) chia seeds
40 g (1½ oz/¼ cup) almonds
30 g (1 oz/⅓ cup) desiccated
    coconut

55 g (2 oz/⅓ cup) sunflower seeds
2 tablespoons peanut butter
1 tablespoon raw cacao powder
1 tablespoon water
toasted shredded coconut,
    for topping

DARK CHOCOLATE + SESAME BLISS BALLS

110 g (3¾ oz/½ cup) pitted
    prunes
80 g (2¾ oz/½ cup) toasted
    almonds
80 g (2¾ oz/½ cup) toasted
    cashews
85 g (3 oz/½ cup) pitted dates
2 tablespoons raw cacao
    powder

40 g (1½ oz/¼ cup) LSA
    (linseed, sunflower seed
    and almond) meal
1 tablespoon chia seeds
grated zest of 1 orange
2 tablespoons water
toasted sesame seeds,
    for topping

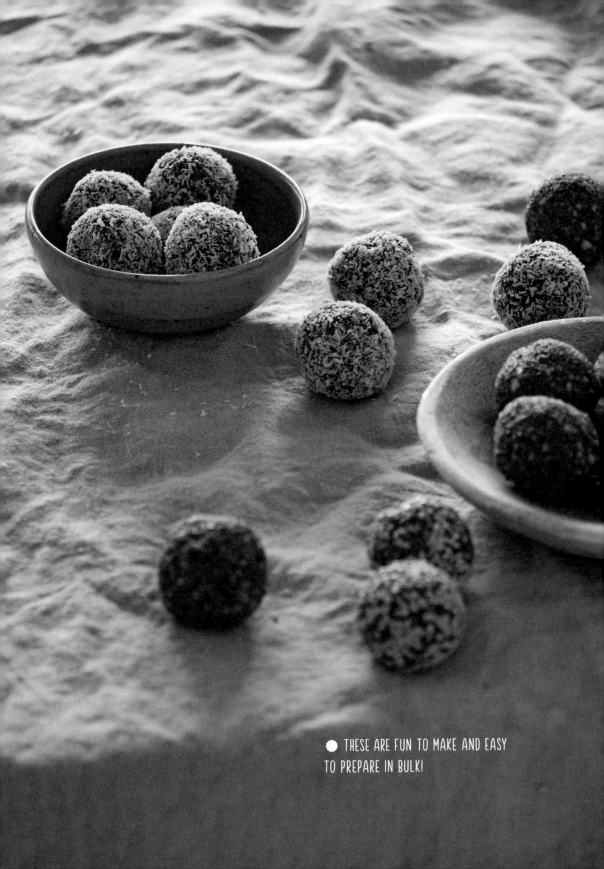

THESE ARE FUN TO MAKE AND EASY TO PREPARE IN BULK!

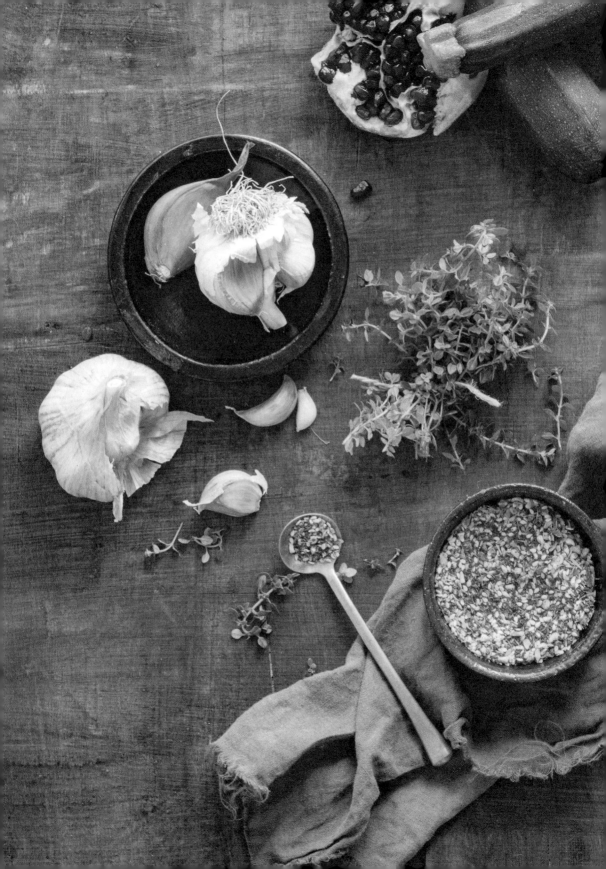

Dinner

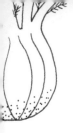

Salmon fishcakes

Fishcakes are an economical way to include more fish in your diet. Tinned salmon is a great way to add more hormone- and mood-friendly omega-3s to your diet and, thanks to the small bones, it's also an excellent source of calcium. I would recommend this recipe if you're avoiding dairy and for those whose menstrual cycles are absent or irregular.

PREPARATION 15 MINS
COOKING 30 MINS
SERVES 4

1 sweet potato, coarsely chopped
2 x 210 g (7½ oz) tins wild-caught salmon with bones, drained
2 eggs, whisked
75 g (2¾ oz/¾ cup) quinoa flakes
½ cup finely chopped fennel
15 g (½ oz/¼ cup) chopped flat-leaf (Italian) parsley
30 g (1 oz/¼ cup) chopped spring onions (scallions)
15 g (½ oz/¼ cup) chopped dill
grated zest of 1 lemon
olive oil, for frying
micro herbs, for serving

Fill a saucepan with water, add the sweet potato and boil for about 10 minutes until soft. Drain and mash with a fork so it cools slightly.

Add the salmon, eggs, quinoa flakes, fennel, parsley spring onion, dill and lemon zest, then season with salt and pepper. Gently mix to combine. Form into small patties roughly the size of the palm of your hand.

Heat a frying pan over medium heat and add olive oil. Fry the patties in the oil until golden on both sides.

Scatter with micro herbs and serve with a green salad, lemon wedges and Creamy tahini dressing (see page 200).

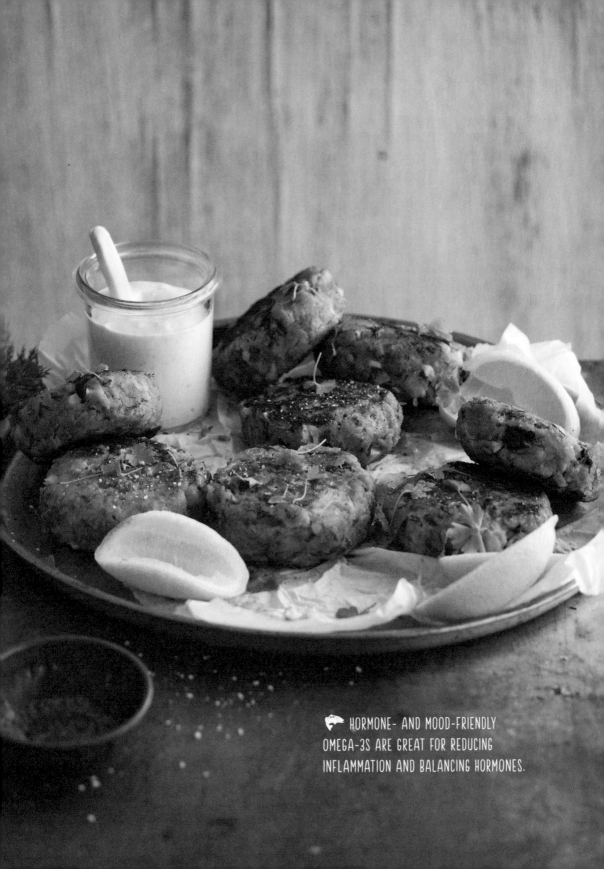

HORMONE- AND MOOD-FRIENDLY
OMEGA-3S ARE GREAT FOR REDUCING
INFLAMMATION AND BALANCING HORMONES.

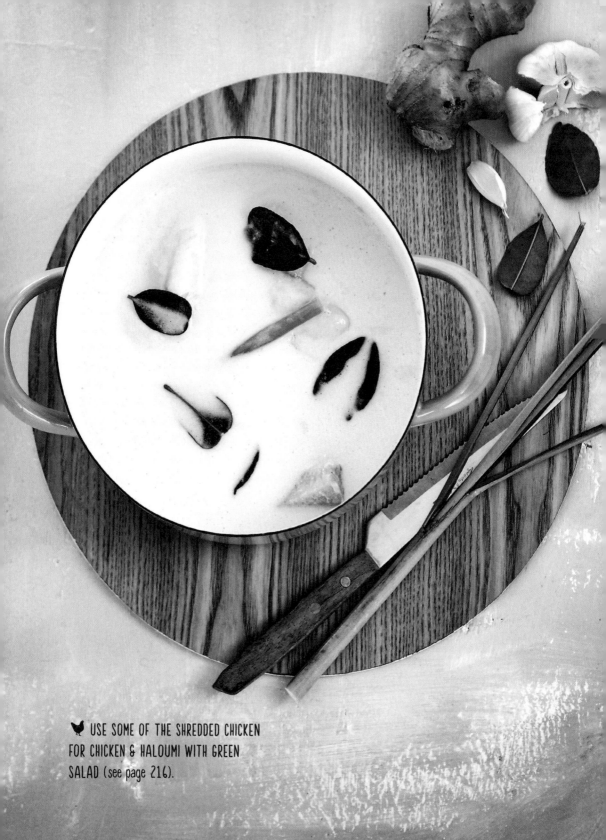

🐓 USE SOME OF THE SHREDDED CHICKEN
FOR CHICKEN & HALOUMI WITH GREEN
SALAD (see page 216).

Creamy coconut chicken

This is the easiest, yummiest chicken that can be served with salads and vegetables or on crackers for lunch. Make a big batch and freeze smaller batches, ready to form the basis of a meal when you're short of time. You can also store chunks of lemongrass, kaffir lime leaves and ginger in the freezer. I always have them on hand! If you make this recipe a day in advance, all the beautiful flavours will intensify. Look for coconut cream that contains only coconuts so that you are not paying for water and other fillers.

PREPARATION 5 MINS
COOKING 20 MINS

1 kg (2 lb 4 oz) boneless chicken breast fillets (about 4 breasts)
2 x 270 ml (9½ fl oz) tins coconut cream
8 cm (3¼ inch) lemongrass stem, crushed
5 kaffir lime leaves
4 cm (1½ inch) piece fresh ginger, coarsely chopped
2 garlic cloves

Put all of the ingredients into a large heavy-based saucepan. Make sure there is enough liquid to cover the chicken: you can top up with water if needed. Bring to the boil, then reduce to a simmer, cover and cook for about 15 minutes or until chicken is cooked through.

Let the chicken rest in the poaching liquid for 5 minutes and then transfer the meat to a container and shred into smaller pieces.

ADD SOME OF THE CREAMY POACHING LIQUID TO THE CONTAINER WITH THE CHICKEN, INCLUDING THE LEMONGRASS, KAFFIR LIME LEAVES AND GINGER. SET ASIDE TO COOL, THEN STORE IN THE FRIDGE READY TO MAKE ASIAN-STYLE LETTUCE CUPS WITH CHICKEN (see page 212).

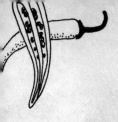

Asian-style lettuce cups
WITH CHICKEN

Tasty, quick and delicious, this recipe is a great crowd pleaser. It can be a little messy and fun to eat using your hands; and it's fresh, light and delicious with the Coconut Chicken. Try making the chicken the day before so the flavour has intensified. If you are avoiding grains, check the health-food store for noodles made from mung beans or kelp. Zucchini noodles are also a great alternative. This is fantastic for lunch if you have leftovers.

PREPARATION 30 MINS
SERVES 3-4

12 cos (romaine) lettuce leaves
vermicelli noodles, softened (optional)
1 Lebanese (short) cucumber, thinly sliced lengthways
1 carrot, thinly sliced lengthways or julienned
1 small handful of snow pea (mangetout) sprouts
1 small handful of bean sprouts
½ red capsicum (pepper), thinly sliced lengthways
½ fresh red chilli, thinly sliced lengthways
1 quantity of Creamy coconut chicken (see page 211)
Asian-style dressing (see page 200)
1 small handful of coriander (cilantro) leaves, for topping
2 tablespoons toasted coconut, for topping
80 g (2¾ oz/½ cup) toasted cashews, for topping

Wash lettuce leaves and spread on a platter. Have all of the remaining ingredients ready to assemble the cups.

Place vermicelli noodles (if using) in each cos leaf then add the salad ingredients. Divide the coconut chicken between the leaves. Drizzle with Asian-style dressing. Top with coriander leaves and sprinkle with toasted coconut and cashews.

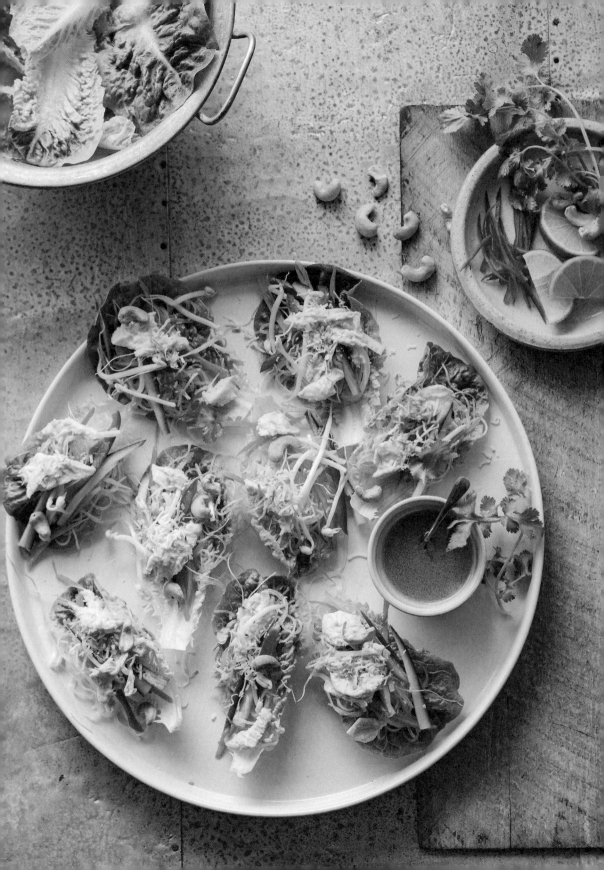

Baked salmon
WITH ZOODLES

There is something really satisfying about making a delicious one-pan dinner: it might be the lack of washing up! This dish is full of hormone-friendly omega-3s and, with the addition of garlic, onion, parsley and oregano, it is also great for those with autoimmune issues. Make zucchini noodles (zoodles) with a small spiralising tool (available from most kitchenware stores) or simply shave the zucchini into long ribbons with your vegetable peeler. Zoodles can be served warmed or raw.

PREPARATION 15 MINS
COOKING 30 MINS
SERVES 4

2 brown onions, cut into small wedges
olive oil, for drizzling
2–3 zucchini (courgettes)
10 cherry tomatoes, halved
10 whole black or green olives, pitted if you prefer
2 garlic cloves, chopped
2 tablespoons oregano leaves
1 handful of flat-leaf (Italian) parsley, chopped
4 salmon fillets
2 tablespoons fig vino cotto
lemon juice, to serve

Preheat the oven to 200°C (400°F).

Put the onions in a large ovenproof baking dish and drizzle with olive oil. Roast the onion for 15 minutes. Meanwhile, spiralise the zucchini and set aside in a bowl.

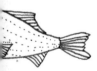

Remove the dish from the oven and reduce the heat to 180°C (350°F). Add the cherry tomatoes, olives, garlic, oregano and parsley to the baking dish and season with salt and pepper.

Place the salmon fillets on the top of the vegetables and drizzle with fig vino cotto. Return to the oven for 15 minutes.

Briefly steam the zucchini for a couple of minutes or cook in the microwave. Divide the zucchini among serving plates, top with the roasted vegetables and place a salmon fillet and some of the roasted herbs on top. Season with salt and pepper.

Squeeze a little lemon juice over each plate.

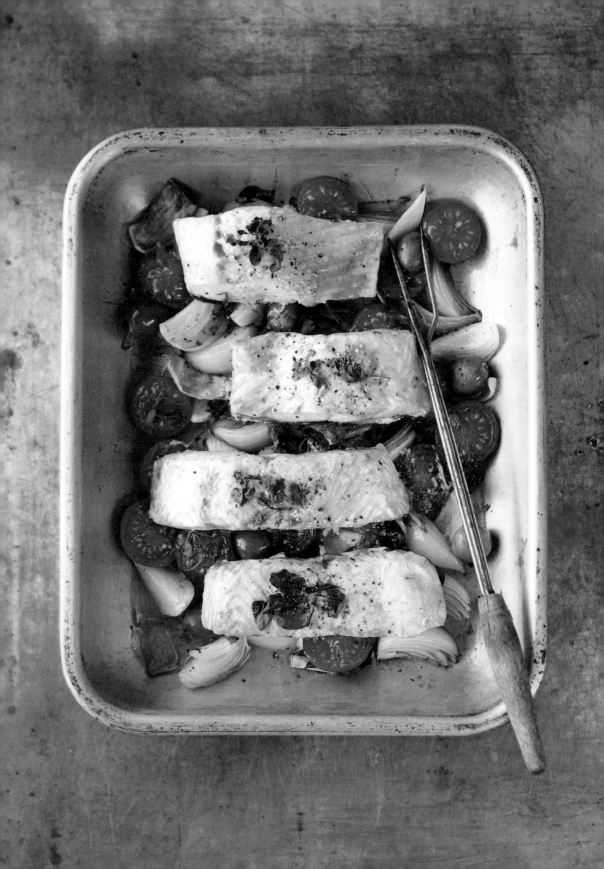

Chicken *and* haloumi
WITH GREEN SALAD

A salad that leaves you satisfied is the best! If you are eating with the family, it can be fun to place a big bowl in the middle of the table for everyone to help themselves. I will often make this with Creamy coconut chicken (see page 211).

PREPARATION 30 MINS
COOKING 10 MINS
SERVES 4

2 boneless chicken breast fillets
10 snow peas (mangetout)
2 tablespoons olive oil
250 g (9 oz) haloumi, sliced into 5 mm (¼ inch) fingers
1 baby cos (romaine) lettuce, leaves sliced in half lengthways
2 zucchini (courgettes), julienned or spiralised
1 Lebanese (short) cucumber, julienned
1 small handful snow pea (mangetout) sprouts
½ avocado, chopped
2 tablespoons sunflower seeds
1 heaped tablespoon coarsely chopped toasted almonds
Green herb dressing (see page 200)

If you don't have any Creamy coconut chicken, poach the chicken in simmering water or coconut cream for about 12 minutes until the chicken is cooked through. Once it has cooled, roughly shred or chop.

Blanch the snow peas in boiling water for 1 minute and then soak in a bowl of icy water to cool. Finely slice lengthways.

Heat 1 tablespoon of olive oil in a frying pan over medium heat and fry the haloumi until brown on each side. Set aside to cool.

In a large serving dish, toss the cos lettuce leaves with the zucchini, cucumber, snow peas, snow pea sprouts and avocado. Add the cooled haloumi and chicken and top with the sunflower seeds and almonds. Season with salt and pepper, then drizzle with plenty of the Green herb dressing.

✗ IF YOU DON'T HAVE ONE, CONSIDER PURCHASING A JULIENNE PEELER: THEY ARE USUALLY CHEAP AND ARE ONE OF THE HANDIEST TOOLS IN THE KITCHEN.

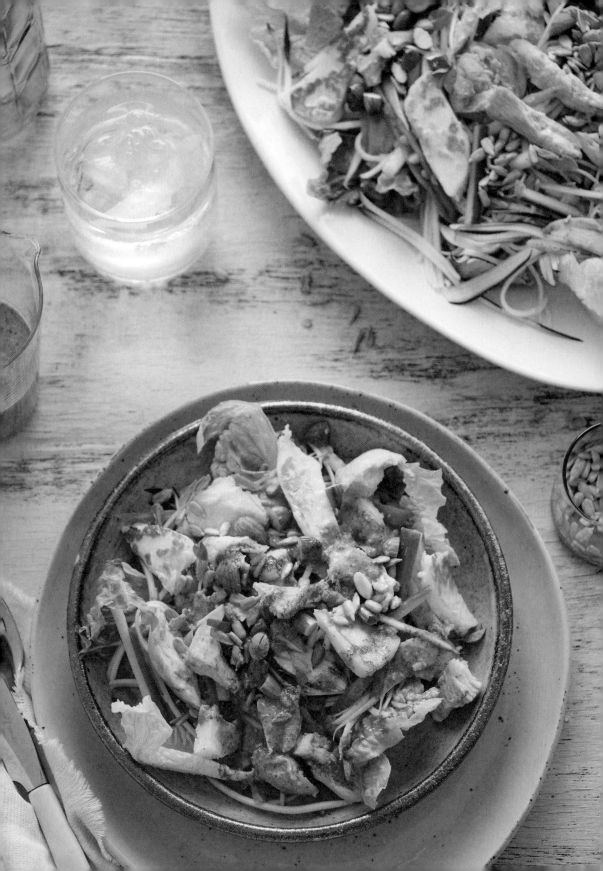

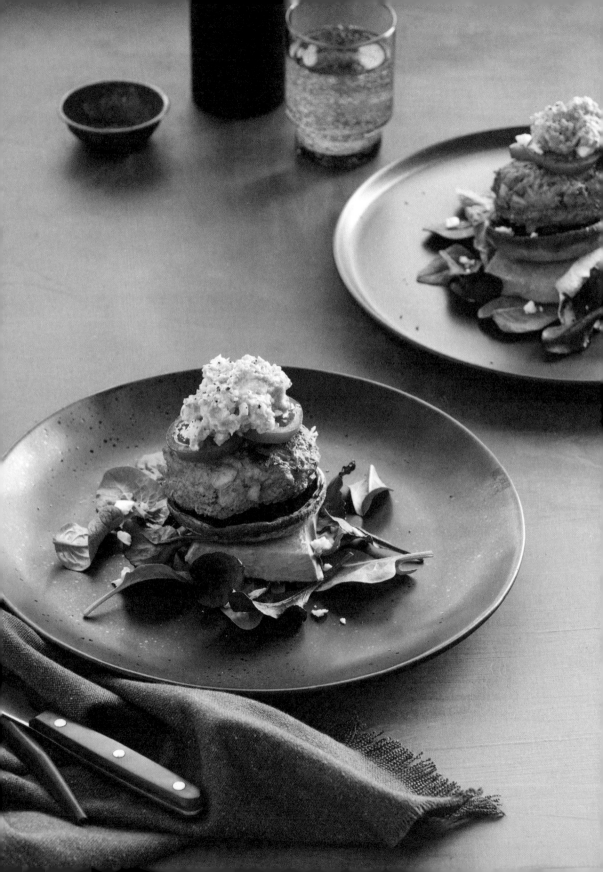

Open burgers

These burgers are an absolute family favourite. Everyone loves a burger; however, white-bread buns and hot chips that they are usually served with make them a less-than-nutritious choice. This recipe gives you all the taste and satisfaction of a burger combined with nutritious sweet-potato chips to balance the meal. Burger patties freeze well so make plenty ahead of time. You can buy ready-made patties from your local butcher (ask what ingredients they use). Once you have had an open burger on a mushroom, you won't even miss the bun!

PREPARATION 15 MINS
COOKING 1 HOUR
SERVES 4

1 large sweet potato sliced lengthways, about 1 cm (⅜ inch) thick
3 tablespoons olive oil
4 large flat mushrooms
500 g (1 lb 2 oz) minced (ground) beef
1 brown onion, chopped
2 tablespoons chopped parsley
1 tablespoon thyme leaves
1 egg, whisked
40 g (1½ oz) baby spinach leaves
1 tomato, sliced
juice of ½ lemon
1 tablespoon crumbled feta cheese
1 avocado, mashed
Creamy tahini dressing (see page 200), optional

Preheat the oven to 200°C (400°F).

Lay the sweet potato slices on a baking tray and drizzle with 2 tablespoons of the olive oil or spray with olive oil spray. Bake for 30 minutes, then reduce oven to 180°C (350°F). Lay the mushrooms on the same tray and bake for a further 20 minutes.

In a bowl, combine beef, onion, parsley, thyme and egg, then season with salt and pepper. Form into 4 burger patties. Heat a large frying pan over medium–high heat, add 1 tablespoon of the olive oil and fry the burger patties for 3–4 minutes on each side, depending on how well done you like them.

To create the burger, place a small handful of spinach leaves on a serving plate, then stack up the sweet potato, mushroom, tomato and feta and top with a good dollop of avocado. Serve with Creamy tahini dressing, if using.

Fish with Asian salad
AND RED CURRY PEA PUREE

This is a great weekend meal as it's a little more fancy and great for entertaining. The red curry pea purée, bursting with a beautiful balance of flavours, makes the dish unique. With such a great range of herbs, it is full of antioxidants and perfect for those trying to conceive or undergoing IVF. Cutting the salad vegetables into matchsticks makes the dish look elegant.

PREPARATION 20 MINS
COOKING 15 MINS
SERVES 4

260 g (9¼ oz/2 cups) frozen baby peas
1–2 teaspoons red curry paste
1 tablespoon sesame oil
1 garlic clove, chopped
1 tablespoon grated fresh ginger
3 cm (1¼ inch) lemongrass stem, very finely sliced
3 kaffir lime leaves, very finely sliced
4 x 180 g (6¼ oz) pieces of firm white-fleshed fish
Asian-style dressing (see page 200)

SALAD

1 large handful of bean sprouts
1 large handful of coriander (cilantro) leaves
1 handful of mint
6–8 snow peas (mangetout), blanched
1 Lebanese (short) cucumber, julienned
½ capsicum (pepper), julienned
½ red chilli, finely sliced
2 tablespoons toasted coconut
40 g (1½ oz/¼ cup) cashews, toasted

Cook the peas in a saucepan of boiling water for about 2 minutes. Drain and transfer to a smoothie maker or blender to blitz until really smooth. Add the red curry paste a teaspoon at a time and mix together until blended. Taste as you add it: the purée shouldn't be too strong — just a nice hint of flavour. Add a tablespoon of water if the purée is too thick.

Heat a medium frying pan over medium heat and stir the sesame oil, garlic, ginger, lemongrass and lime leaves for a few minutes. Move the mixture to the side of the pan and add the fish. Spoon the herb mix onto the fish while it is cooking. Cook fish for about 5–8 minutes depending on the size, until it is just cooked through.

To make the salad, combine the bean sprouts, coriander, mint, snow peas, cucumber and capsicum in a bowl. Mix well, then top with chilli, toasted coconut, toasted cashews. Dress with some of the Asian-style dressing.

To serve, place a large spoonful of pea purée on each plate, top with a piece of fish and add some salad on the side.

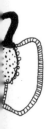

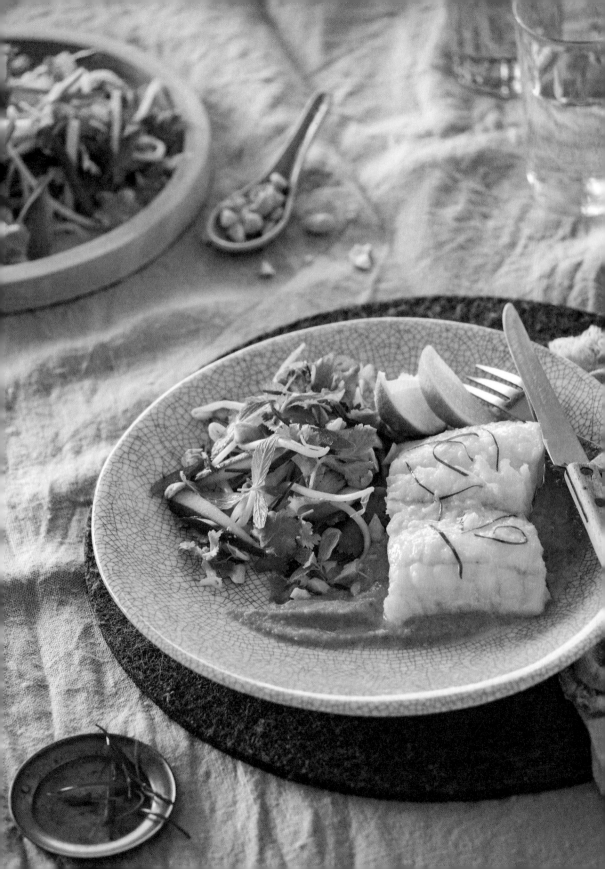

Quinoa-crusted chicken
WITH CHICKPEA SALAD

This recipe is a nutritious version of fried chicken. Coated in quinoa and almond meal instead of breadcrumbs, these chicken pieces are great for supporting oestrogen metabolism and a good choice for those suffering from PMS, period pain or fatigue. You can serve these with hummus, pesto, guacamole or Creamy tahini dressing (see page 200) in addition to the chickpea salad. Cook extra quinoa so that you can use some for this recipe and use the leftovers to make the Quinoa salad (see page 193) for lunch.

PREPARATION 20 MINS
COOKING 10 MINS
SERVES 3-4

¾ cup cooked quinoa
1 tablespoon milk
1 tablespoon chopped flat-leaf (Italian) parsley
1 egg, whisked
2 tablespoons almond meal
500–600 g (1 lb 2 oz–1 lb 5 oz) skinless boneless chicken thighs, halved
olive oil, for frying
Creamy tahini dressing (see page 200)

CHICKPEA SALAD

400 g (14 oz) tin chickpeas (garbanzo beans) or 70 g (2½ oz/⅓ cup) dried chickpeas, soaked and boiled
2 corn cobs, blanched and kernels removed
½ Lebanese (short) cucumber, chopped
10–12 cherry tomatoes, finely chopped
1 French shallot, finely chopped
1 tablespoon chopped mint
½ avocado, chopped
Green herb dressing (see page 200)

Combine quinoa, milk, parsley, egg and almond meal in a bowl and season with salt and pepper. This is a mixture that is soft and easy to form. Mould an amount to roughly fit the chicken piece and carefully press onto one side of the chicken (the smooth side is easiest). Repeat until all the chicken is covered.

Heat olive oil in a non-stick frying pan over medium–high heat. Place the chicken pieces quinoa side down and fry for 3–4 minutes until golden and crisp. Carefully flip over and cook the other side for a further 2–3 minutes until cooked through. You can cook them in batches and place them in a moderate oven until they are all done.

To make the chickpea salad, combine all of the ingredients in a bowl and drizzle with the Green herb dressing. Season with salt and pepper.

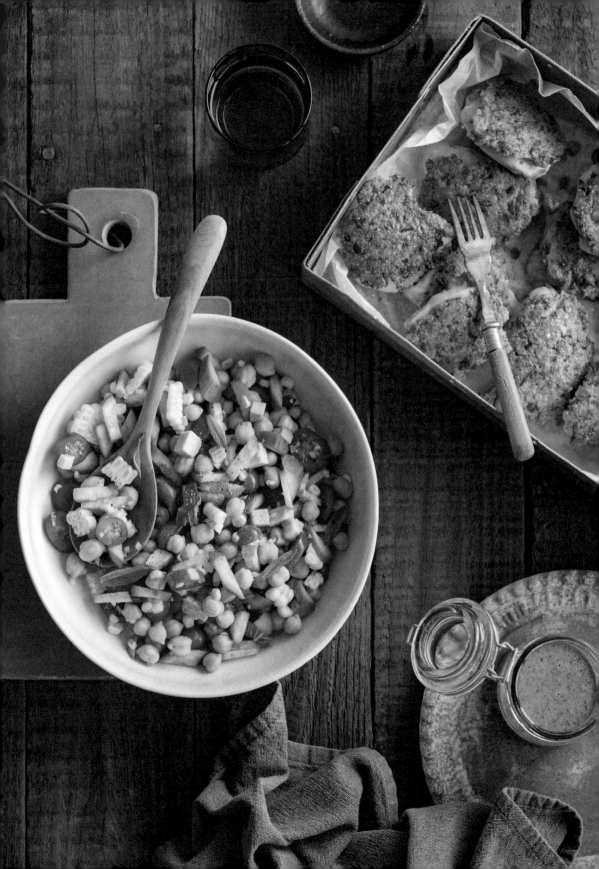

Simple roast lamb and veggies

Who doesn't love a lamb roast? It's super-easy and very satisfying. If you haven't tried roasted brussels sprouts before, now is the time. This recipe is sure to convert the majority of 'sprout-haters'. Roasting ensures that the sprouts are sweet and tasty. The nutrient-dense sprouts are high in fibre, high in vitamins A and C, immune boosting and essential for those with relative oestrogen excess. If you have ovarian cysts, polyps, heavy periods or low mood, this recipe is especially for you! Remember to save some for lunch the next day. You can pop some of the roast lamb on seed crackers with hummus, sliced cucumber and tomatoes: delish!

PREPARATION 20 MINS

COOKING 1 HOUR 15 MINS

SERVES 4

125 g (4½ oz/½ cup) pitted black olives, coarsely chopped
3 garlic cloves, chopped
2 tablespoons finely chopped rosemary
2 tablespoons thyme leaves
2 tablespoons extra virgin olive oil
1.5 kg (3 lb 5 oz) lamb leg
400 g (14 oz) brussels sprouts, halved
4–5 baby sweet potatoes, halved
4 onions, halved
6–8 carrots, halved lengthways
1 tablespoon dukkah
Creamy tahini dressing (see page 200), to serve

Preheat the oven to 180°C (350°F).

Mix together olives, garlic, rosemary and thyme with 1 tablespoon of the olive oil and season with salt and pepper.

Put the lamb in a roasting tin and spoon the olive and herb mixture over the top. Don't worry if some falls off, it will all get mixed in with the pan juices.

Line a baking tray with foil and spread with the chopped vegetables. Drizzle a small amount of olive oil over them.

Roast the lamb for 1 hour 15 minutes for medium-rare. The general rule for cooking lamb roasts is 25–30 minutes per 500 g (1 lb 2 oz). Put the tray of vegetables into the oven 40 minutes before cooking time is up.

To serve, carve the lamb into slices. Transfer the roasted vegetables to a serving dish and sprinkle with the dukkah. Serve with Creamy tahini dressing.

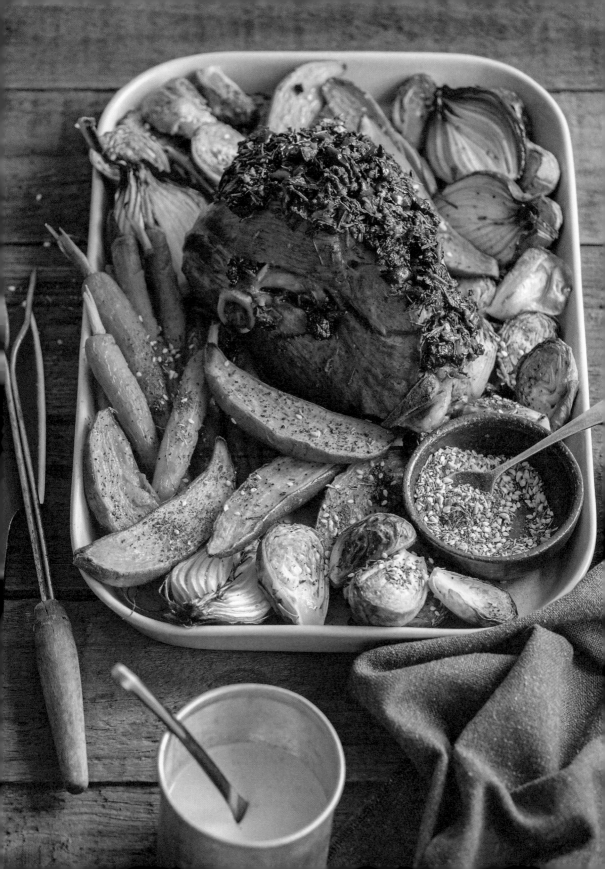

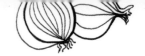

Moroccan beef

This easy one-pot dinner is a warm, hearty meal that can be made in the oven or your slow cooker. Moroccan beef has a mildly spicy flavour and is suitable for the whole family. Slow-cooking can make red meat easier to digest, making this dish perfect for those with a sluggish digestive system. Ras el hanout is a Moroccan spice mix that is usually available in the supermarket.

PREPARATION 25 MINS
COOKING 2-3 HOURS
SERVES 4

1 tablespoon olive oil
1 kg (2 lb 4 oz) beef (chuck, gravy beef, shin or round steak) cut into 2.5 cm (1 inch) cubes
2 onions, cut into wedges
3 garlic cloves, chopped
grated zest and juice of 1 orange
1 tablespoon dried parsley
1 tablespoon dried coriander
1 tablespoon thyme leaves
2 tablespoons ras el hanout or Moroccan spice mix
3 carrots, cut into 4 cm (1½ inch) chunks
130 g (4½ oz) pitted dates, coarsely chopped
410 g (14½ oz) tin tomatoes
140 g (5 oz) tomato paste (concentrated purée)
400 g (14 oz) tin chickpeas (garbanzo beans) or 70 g (2½ oz/⅓ cup) dried chickpeas, soaked and boiled
1 handful of flat-leaf (Italian) parsley, coarsely chopped
Plain yoghurt, mint leaves and roasted almonds, to serve
Cooked quinoa, to serve

Heat the olive oil in a heavy-based saucepan over medium–high heat, add the beef and season with salt and pepper. Brown all over for a couple of minutes.

Add the onion, garlic, orange zest and juice, herbs and spices. Stir well so the beef is coated.

Add the carrots, dates, tomatoes, tomato paste, chickpeas and 2 tomato tins (about 800 ml/28 fl oz) of water and stir. Bring to the boil, then reduce to a simmer and cook for 2–3 hours until the beef is very tender. Add the chopped fresh parsley.

To serve, divide among plates and top with yoghurt, mint leaves and roasted almonds. Serve with the cooked quinoa.

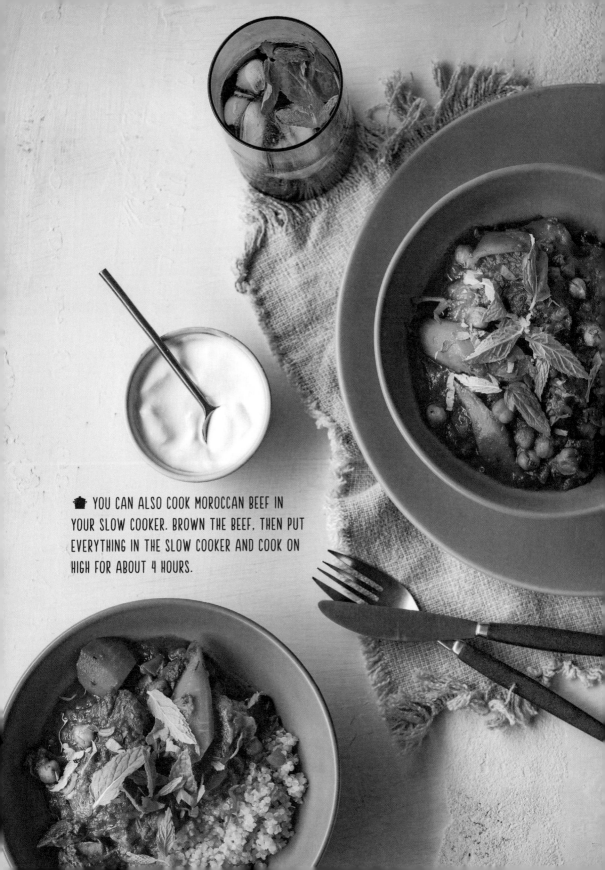

YOU CAN ALSO COOK MOROCCAN BEEF IN YOUR SLOW COOKER. BROWN THE BEEF, THEN PUT EVERYTHING IN THE SLOW COOKER AND COOK ON HIGH FOR ABOUT 4 HOURS.

Strawberry chia puddings

Chia seeds are amazing for increasing satiety (so you feel fuller and don't eat as much). They also balance blood-sugar levels, improve sluggish bowels, improve energy levels and provide a yummy dessert, a great school or work lunch box snack or a quick breakfast. Chia seed puddings are incredibly forgiving and can be made by anyone!

PREPARATION 5 MINS
SERVES 2

250 g (9 oz) strawberries
40 g (1½ oz/¼ cup) chia seeds
125 g (4½ oz/½ cup) coconut cream
2 teaspoons vanilla paste
2 teaspoons raw cacao nibs, for topping
4 brazil nuts, coarsely chopped, for topping
1 white nectarine, sliced

Wash and hull the strawberries and put them in a bowl with 1 tablespoon of water. Transfer to a smoothie maker or use a handheld blender to blitz until smooth.

Put the chia seeds, coconut cream, 125 ml (4 fl oz/½ cup) of the strawberry purée, 125 ml (4 fl oz/½ cup) of water and vanilla paste in a bowl and stir until well combined. Leave in the fridge for at least 15 minutes until all the ingredients have come together and the chia seeds have swollen.

When ready to eat, spoon the chia pudding into bowls or glasses. Top with some of the remaining strawberry purée, cacao nibs, chopped brazil nuts and a few slices of the white nectarine.

★ IF YOU FIND THE MIXTURE IS TOO RUNNY, ADD MORE CHIA SEEDS AND POP IT BACK IN THE FRIDGE FOR 10 MINUTES. IF THE PUDDING IS TOO HARD, JUST ADD MORE LIQUID AND IN 10 MINUTES THE PUDDING WILL BE THE RIGHT CONSISTENCY.

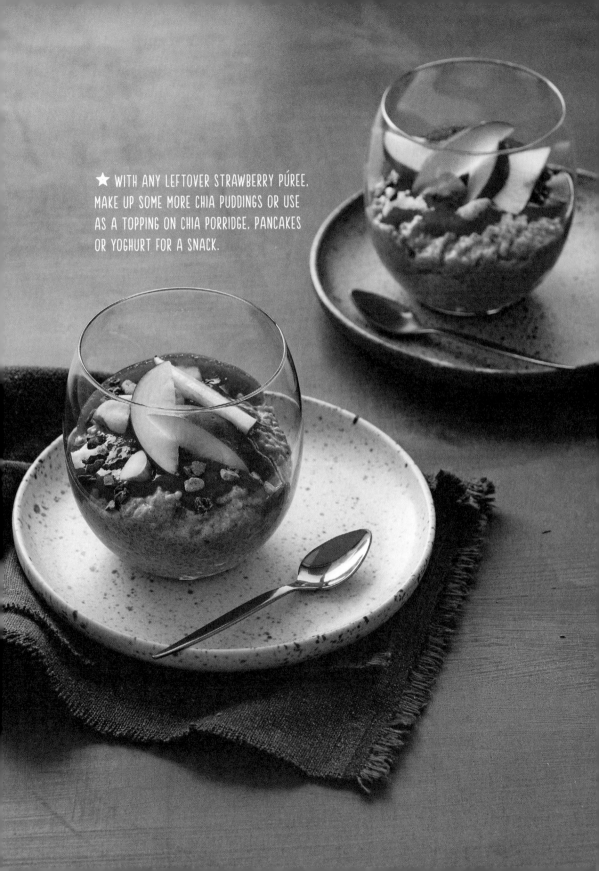

★ WITH ANY LEFTOVER STRAWBERRY PÚREE, MAKE UP SOME MORE CHIA PUDDINGS OR USE AS A TOPPING ON CHIA PORRIDGE, PANCAKES OR YOGHURT FOR A SNACK.

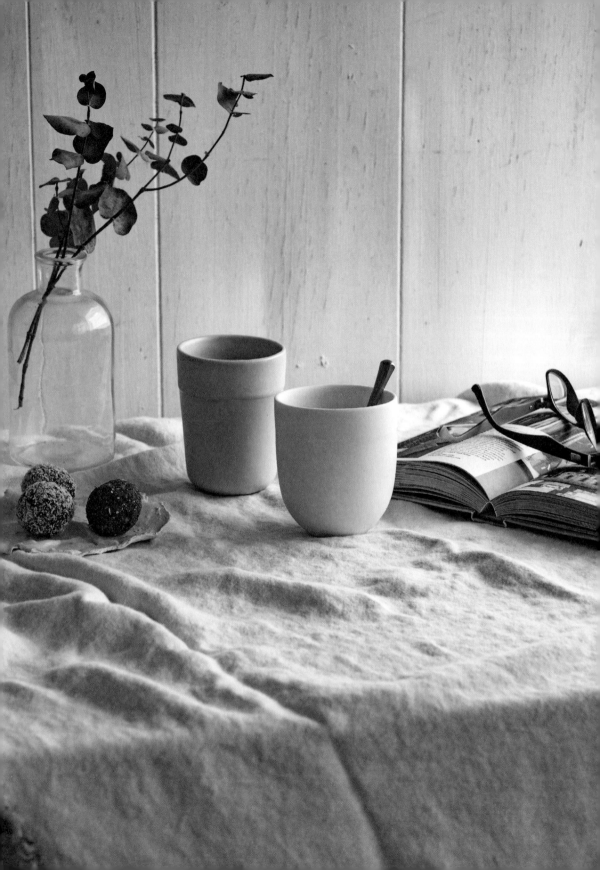

Turmeric chai

This warming drink is a caffeine-free alternative to coffee and the perfect hot drink for when you need more than just herbal tea after dinner. The combination of warming spices is great for digestion and circulation and is especially created to be consumed while you have your period to help support flow and reduce cramps.

PREPARATION 5 MINS
COOKING 5 MINS
SERVES 2

60 ml (2 fl oz/¼ cup) coconut milk
125 ml (4½ fl oz/½ cup) almond milk
60 ml (2 fl oz/¼ cup) water
1 teaspoon ground turmeric
1 teaspoon ground cinnamon
pinch of black pepper
1 star anise
3 cardamom pods
4 cm (1½ inch) piece of orange peel
1 teaspoon honey

Put all of the ingredients into a saucepan and stir over medium heat for about 5 minutes.

Strain and serve in mugs.

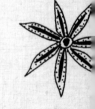

SUPPLEMENTS

MORE INFORMATION It's best if a naturopath prescribes supplements so they can ensure you are taking everything you need (and nothing you don't); indicate how long you should take the supplement for; and ensure there are no contraindications. Always mention any supplements you are taking to your doctor to make sure there are no conflicts or potential interactions with prescription medicines.

CALCIUM

Calcium is involved in muscle contraction and relaxation and is useful for premenstrual cramping and endometriosis. Calcium is useful for treating PMS symptoms of irritability, fluid retention, depression and fatigue. Calcium is also essential for healthy bones with requirements increasing at menopause to prevent osteoporosis.

WHO MIGHT NEED IT? Calcium supplementation may be useful for those with low dietary intake of calcium or dairy products, women experiencing PMS, perimenopausal and menopausal women, pregnant and lactating women.

WHAT TO LOOK FOR: Look for supplements containing calcium hydroxyapatite, calcium citrate or calcium phosphate as these are absorbed well by the body. Avoid calcium carbonate, as this form does not absorb well in the body. Calcium is best taken with a meal.

DAILY DOSAGE YOUR NATUROPATH MIGHT RECOMMEND: Daily dosage should be calculated based on deficiency and excess calcium is not recommended. It is ideal to calculate daily calcium intake and then make up the rest with a supplement if food sources cannot be regularly consumed. Dose would usually be around 500mg of calcium and is best taken with breakfast.

FOOD SOURCES INCLUDE: Milk; yoghurt; cheese; tinned salmon with bones; tinned sardines with bones; almonds; sesame seeds; tahini; green leafy vegetables.

CHROMIUM

Chromium helps to control blood-sugar levels as well as the metabolism of protein and fat. It is useful for PCOS, insulin resistance, diabetes and metabolic syndrome.

WHO MIGHT NEED IT? Those with insulin resistance, sugar cravings or who consume high amounts of carbohydrate foods may benefit from taking chromium supplementation.

WHAT TO LOOK FOR: The best form to look for is chromium picolinate as it absorbs well in the body. Chromium is best taken just before a meal.

DAILY DOSAGE YOUR NATUROPATH MIGHT RECOMMEND: PCOS: 1000mcg; Insulin resistance: 200–1000mcg

FOOD SOURCES INCLUDE: Parsley; spinach; apples; red meat; oysters; asparagus; mushrooms; cheese; prunes; raisins.

COENZYME Q10

Coenzyme Q10 (CoQ10) plays an important role in energy production and is a potent antioxidant. CoQ10 is necessary for healthy egg production and ovulation. It can help support conception by promoting better quality eggs and embryos.

WHO MIGHT NEED IT? Supplementation is recommended for women wanting to conceive, especially women over the age of 35. Supplementation is also useful for those with fatigue, low immunity and those wanting to improve exercise performance.

WHAT TO LOOK FOR: There are two forms of CoQ10, Ubiquinone and Ubiquinol. Ubiquinone is recommended for active people with general good health, whereas ubiquinol is recommended for people with suboptimal health or women over the age of 35 wanting to conceive. CoQ10 is best taken with meals containing a fat.

DAILY DOSAGE YOUR NATUROPATH MIGHT RECOMMEND: Preconception: 300mg; Fatigue: 150–300mg; IVF support: 400mg

FOOD SOURCES INCLUDE: Beef; almonds; broccoli; mackerel; sardines; salmon; sesame seeds.

FOLATE

Folate is useful in conditions where there is oestrogen excess, including endometriosis, uterine fibroids, heavy periods, breast cysts, ovarian cysts and breast pain. Folate supplementation is also essential during pregnancy and for at least three months prior to conception. Folate can help reduce neural tube defects, miscarriage, autism, depression and pre-eclampsia. See page 65 for more information about folate.

WHO MIGHT NEED IT? Those with a genetic mutation that affects folate metabolism may require supplementation. Women who have heavy periods and those taking the oral contraceptive pill may also benefit from folate supplementation, as well as women wanting to conceive.

WHAT TO LOOK FOR: The best form to look for is folinic acid or methyl-tetrahydrofolate. These forms are more easily utilised by the body. If you have the genetic mutation that affects folate metabolism it is important that you avoid synthetic folic acid and only take the methyl-tetrahydrofolate or folinic acid form.

DAILY DOSAGE YOUR NATUROPATH MIGHT RECOMMEND: Preconception and pregnancy: 600mcg
Recurrent miscarriage and MTHFR mutations may require a tailored dose.

FOOD SOURCES INCLUDE: Green leafy vegetables; lentils; eggs; mung beans; adzuki beans.

INDOLE-3-CARBINOL (I-3-C) / 3,3-DIINDOLYMETHANE (DIM)

Indole-3-Carbinol (I-3-C) and 3,3-diindolymethane (DIM) are compounds found in brassica vegetables (broccoli, cabbage, kale, cauliflower, brussels sprouts). They help eliminate excess oestrogen and may reduce the risk of breast and cervical cancer.

WHO MIGHT NEED IT? I-3-C or DIM are very useful in women with endometriosis and conditions of relative oestrogen excess. Women with a family history of breast or cervical cancer may also benefit from taking this supplement.

WHAT TO LOOK FOR: Indole-3-Carbinol is available as Indole-3-Carbinol (I-3-C) or as 3,3-diindolymethane (DIM). Use of this supplement is best supervised by a practitioner. It should be taken with food.

DAILY DOSAGE YOUR NATUROPATH MIGHT RECOMMEND: DIM = 100–300mg OR I-3-C = 400–800mg

FOOD SOURCES INCLUDE: Broccoli; cabbage; cauliflower; kale; brussels sprouts.

INOSITOL

Inositol may help to increase progesterone and is useful in conditions of low progesterone, including short cycles, premenstrual spotting and PMS. Inositol increases the action of insulin and is effective in PCOS, restoring insulin sensitivity, reducing acne and excess hair growth, in addition to restoring normal menstrual cycling and fertility. Inositol is also used in Hashimoto's thyroiditis (often in combination with selenium) to reduce elevated TSH and antibodies.

WHO MIGHT NEED IT? Those with PCOS, hypothyroidism, experiencing stress, low mood or anxiety may benefit from taking inositol supplementation.

WHAT TO LOOK FOR: Inositol is best taken as myo-inositol.

DAILY DOSAGE YOUR NATUROPATH MIGHT RECOMMEND: 300–1000mg

FOOD SOURCES INCLUDE: Rockmelon; citrus fruits; sweet corn; lentils; haricot (navy) beans.

IODINE

Iodine is useful for treating heavy periods, breast cysts, ovarian cysts, uterine fibroids, endometriosis and breast pain. Iodine is also used to make thyroid hormones and requirements are increased during pregnancy.

WHO MIGHT NEED IT? Many people are iodine deficient, particularly those who do not eat seafood, seaweed or salt.

WHAT TO LOOK FOR: The safest form to look for is potassium iodide. Iodine should be taken with food to enhance absorption. Never take iodine supplements without supervision from a practitioner as iodine may aggravate thyroid disease in some people (for example, those with hyperthyroidism, Graves' disease or who are taking thyroxine).

DAILY DOSAGE YOUR NATUROPATH MIGHT RECOMMEND: It is important to test for iodine deficiency and supplement according to your deficiency because oversupplementation can be dangerous.

FOOD SOURCES INCLUDE: Kelp; seaweed; clams; prawns; oysters; salmon; cod; snapper.

IRON

Iron is used in conditions where there is blood loss, including heavy periods, endometriosis and uterine fibroids. It is also essential for proper thyroid and immune function and is important in pregnancy.

WHO MIGHT NEED IT? Women who experience heavy menstrual blood loss, vegetarians and vegans may benefit from iron supplementation.

WHAT TO LOOK FOR: The best form to look for is iron bisglycinate or iron picolinate, which is a highly absorbable form of iron and gentle on the stomach. Iron is best taken after a meal containing vitamin C, such as broccoli, capsicum (peppers), tomatoes.

DAILY DOSAGE YOUR NATUROPATH MIGHT RECOMMEND: Iron can be inflammatory and can be harmful in excess. It is important to test for iron levels and supplement only according to your deficiency. Iron is contraindicated in haemochromatosis.

FOOD SOURCES INCLUDE: Red meat; eggs; lentils; parsley; spinach; pine nuts; pepitas (pumpkin seeds); sunflower seeds.

LIPOIC ACID

Lipoic acid is a potent antioxidant that is useful in treating PCOS as it can help improve glucose metabolism and insulin sensitivity. As an antioxidant, lipoic acid also helps to prepare your body for conception.

WHO MIGHT NEED IT? Women with PCOS and those wanting to conceive.

WHAT TO LOOK FOR: The best form to look for is R,S-alpha lipoic acid. It is recommended to take lipoic acid on an empty stomach to improve bioavailability.

DAILY DOSAGE YOUR NATUROPATH MIGHT RECOMMEND: PCOS: 300–600mg; Women over 35 trying to conceive: 400–800mg

FOOD SOURCES INCLUDE: Broccoli; Brussels sprouts; organ meats; potatoes; spinach; tomatoes.

MAGNESIUM

Magnesium helps to relax muscles and calm the nervous system. It is used for period pain, endometriosis, PMS, headaches, stress, anxiety, insomnia and constipation. Magnesium can also help with insulin resistance, so is used to help with PCOS.

WHO MIGHT NEED IT? Anyone who is experiencing stress may benefit from taking a magnesium supplement, as stress can increase the depletion of magnesium from the body. Magnesium is also essential for those experiencing muscle cramps, poor sleep, fatigue and relative progesterone deficiency.

WHAT TO LOOK FOR: The best forms to look for are magnesium citrate or magnesium glycinate as they absorb well in the body. Avoid magnesium oxide, as this form does not absorb well in the body and may cause loose stools. Magnesium is best taken in the morning for increased energy or just before bed to promote a restful sleep.

DAILY DOSAGE YOUR NATUROPATH MIGHT RECOMMEND: Endometriosis: 500–1000mg; PCOS: 500–1000mg; PMS: 400–800mg; Period pain: 300–600mg

FOOD SOURCES INCLUDE: Green leafy vegetables; almonds; cashews; pepitas (pumpkin seeds); linseeds (flaxseeds); parsley; brazil nuts; tahini.

NAC (N-ACETYL CYSTEINE)

NAC is an antioxidant. It is anti-inflammatory and helps promote detoxification. NAC is used for endometriosis, PCOS, to improve ovulation and support pregnancy. NAC may also be recommended for detoxification, allergies, respiratory infections and addictions.

WHO MIGHT NEED IT? Women with endometriosis, PCOS and those wanting to conceive may benefit from taking NAC. Those suffering from low immunity, chronic respiratory infections, allergies and addictions may also benefit.

DAILY DOSAGE YOUR NATUROPATH MIGHT RECOMMEND: Endometriosis: 600mg three times daily; PCOS: 500–1000mg; IVF support: 600mg twice daily

OMEGA-3

The anti-inflammatory effect of omega–3 (e.g. fish oils) can help to balance hormones, reduce pain and inflammation. These actions are useful for PMS, heavy periods, failure to get a period, irregular periods, short cycles, endometriosis and uterine fibroids. Fish oils are also used in PCOS to help regulate blood glucose levels.

WHO MIGHT NEED IT? Omega–3 supplementation is recommended for people who do not eat fish and is also essential for anyone suffering from inflammation, pain or autoimmunity. Conditions which fish oils are beneficial for include: pregnancy; breastfeeding; eczema; asthma; allergies; autoimmune diseases; anxiety; depression; PMS; painful periods; heavy periods; no periods; endometriosis; uterine fibroids; PCOS; acne.

WHAT TO LOOK FOR: Fish oils are available in both capsules and liquid form. Some liquid forms have a higher concentration of EPA and DHA (the active components of omega–3) which may provide better results. When choosing a capsule, look for one with a minimum of 400mg EPA and 200mg DHA. You usually get what you pay for: cheaper products may not be processed as carefully, which may result in them becoming pro-inflammatory instead of anti-inflammatory. Always choose a practitioner-only brand as these are usually third-party tested for purity and efficacy. These brands will also purify the product from any pesticides, persistent organic pollutants and heavy metals that can have detrimental effects on your health. It is usually worth spending the extra money for good quality. Fish oils are best taken with a meal containing a fat.

DAILY DOSAGE YOUR NATUROPATH MIGHT RECOMMEND: Pre-conception: 4000mg; Period pain or hormonal regulation: between 4000 and 6000mg; Endometriosis: 8–10,000mg; Uterine fibroids: 3000mg

FOOD SOURCES INCLUDE: Salmon; tuna; trout; mackerel; sardines; chia seeds; linseeds (flaxseeds).

PROBIOTICS

Probiotics help to maintain healthy intestinal bacteria, which can promote oestrogen elimination. Probiotics are useful in conditions of relative oestrogen excess, including endometriosis, uterine fibroids, heavy periods, breast cysts, ovarian cysts and breast pain. Probiotics are also useful for digestive complaints, poor immunity and recurrent thrush.

WHO MIGHT NEED IT? People with a low intake of fibre, those who have been on antibiotics and those with chronic low immunity or digestive issues may benefit from taking a probiotic.

WHAT TO LOOK FOR: Aim to choose a product that has multiple strains to ensure you don't overpopulate your gut with just one strain. Rotate the type of probiotic that you use to promote a healthy balance of different strains of bacteria. Look for beneficial strains including *Lactobacillus acidophilus*, *L. plantarum*, *L. rhamnosus*, *Bifidobacterium animalis* subsp. *lactis* and *B. longum*.

DAILY DOSAGE YOUR NATUROPATH MIGHT RECOMMEND: Take 1 capsule or 1 teaspoon (minimum 30 billion bacteria) before breakfast daily.

FOOD SOURCES INCLUDE: Yoghurt; sauerkraut; kefir; kombucha; miso.

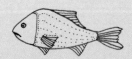

SELENIUM

Selenium helps with progesterone production and may be useful in conditions of relative progesterone deficiency, including short cycles, premenstrual spotting and PMS. Selenium also assists with the elimination of oestrogen from the body and is therefore useful in conditions of relative oestrogen excess, including uterine fibroids, endometriosis, heavy periods, breast cysts, ovarian cysts and breast pain. Selenium is also required for normal thyroid and immune function, can reduce thyroid antibodies and is an antioxidant.

WHO MIGHT NEED IT? Selenium is very low in Australian soil, which means that deficiency is common. It is important to note that selenium can be toxic at high levels so it is important not to take more than the recommended dose.

WHAT TO LOOK FOR: The best form to look for is selenomethionine as it is very well absorbed in the body.

DAILY DOSAGE YOUR NATUROPATH MIGHT RECOMMEND: 100–150mcg

FOOD SOURCES INCLUDE: Brazil nuts; shellfish; fish; eggs; tinned salmon; tinned sardines; cashews.

VITAMIN B6

Vitamin B6 is useful for almost all symptoms of PMS including fluid retention, cramping, anxiety, depression and insomnia.

WHO MIGHT NEED IT? Anyone who is experiencing stress may benefit from taking a vitamin B6 supplement.

WHAT TO LOOK FOR: Pyridoxine hydrochloride (inactive form) is the most common supplemental form of vitamin B6. Its active form is Pyridoxal-5-Phosphate or P-5-P. Pyridoxal-5-Phosphate is the preferred form as it is the form the body uses. Vitamin B6 is best taken with a meal.

DAILY DOSAGE YOUR NATUROPATH MIGHT RECOMMEND: PMS: 25–50mg

FOOD SOURCES INCLUDE: Sunflower seeds; walnuts; brown rice; pistachio nuts; hazelnuts; lentils; chickpeas (garbanzo beans); eggs.

VITAMIN B12

Vitamin B12 can help clear oestrogen from the body; it is therefore useful in conditions where there is oestrogen excess, including endometriosis, uterine fibroids, heavy periods, breast cysts, ovarian cysts and breast pain.

WHO MIGHT NEED IT? Vegetarians and vegans will benefit from taking vitamin B12 as it is only found in adequate amounts in animal foods. Women with heavy periods may also benefit from B12 supplementation.

WHAT TO LOOK FOR: Cyanocobalamin is the most common supplemental form of vitamin B12. The best form is methyl-cobalamin. Vitamin B12 is available in sublingual oral preparations or sprays, which are easily absorbed by the body.

DAILY DOSAGE YOUR NATUROPATH MIGHT RECOMMEND: Vegans and vegetarians: minimum of 300mcg with breakfast; Pre-conception: 400–1000mcg

FOOD SOURCES INCLUDE: Salmon; sardines; herring; eggs; oysters; red meat.

VITAMIN C

Vitamin C is a potent antioxidant useful in conditions of oxidative stress, including endometriosis and PCOS. Vitamin C is also an immune stimulant useful in conditions such as pelvic inflammatory disease, vaginitis, as well as colds, influenza and respiratory tract infections. Vitamin C also helps maintain healthy ovarian function.

WHO MIGHT NEED IT? People with low immune function (recurrent colds and flu), those who consume minimal fresh fruit and vegetables, and those experiencing stress may benefit from taking a vitamin C supplement. Vitamin C is also beneficial for older women trying to conceive and those doing IVF.

WHAT TO LOOK FOR: Look for vitamin C as calcium ascorbate or magnesium ascorbate as these forms are nonacidic and better tolerated by the stomach. Vitamin C is better taken in small doses and often. If loose bowels result, reduce the amount you are taking.

DAILY DOSAGE YOUR NATUROPATH MIGHT RECOMMEND: 500–3000mg daily in divided doses.

FOOD SOURCES INCLUDE: Red capsicum (pepper); broccoli; kiwifruit; mango; strawberries; parsley; citrus fruits.

VITAMIN D

Vitamin D is a hormone precursor essential for progesterone production. Conditions of low progesterone include short menstrual cycles, premenstrual spotting and PMS. Vitamin D also improves insulin sensitivity in PCOS, and is important for immunity, bone health and balanced mood.

WHO MIGHT NEED IT? Vitamin D increases with sun exposure, therefore people who spend little time in the sun and those who cover exposed skin with sunscreen or clothes may need supplementation. People with dark skin may also require vitamin D supplementation.

WHAT TO LOOK FOR: The best form to look for is vitamin D3, known as cholecalciferol. This is the form your body makes when it is exposed to the sun. Vitamin D should be taken with a meal to help absorption.

DAILY DOSAGE YOUR NATUROPATH MIGHT RECOMMEND: It is important to test for vitamin D levels and supplement according to your deficiency. Up to 5000IU per day may be required for hormonal health when vitamin D levels are low.

FOOD SOURCES INCLUDE: Organic butter; sardines; egg yolks.

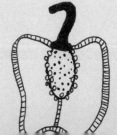

VITAMIN E

Vitamin E is a potent antioxidant and anti-inflammatory nutrient that helps balance hormones. It is useful for PMS, breast pain, endometriosis, PCOS, pelvic inflammatory disease and helps maintain healthy ovaries. Vitamin E is also used to promote healthy skin and improve wound healing.

WHO MIGHT NEED IT? Women with relative oestrogen deficiency, thin uterine lining or scanty bleeds in addition to older women trying to conceive and those undergoing IVF.

WHAT TO LOOK FOR: Natural vitamin E occurs as a family of eight different compounds: four tocopherols and four tocotrienols. Ideally look for a supplement that contains a mixture of both. Vitamin E should be taken with a meal to help absorption.

DAILY DOSAGE YOUR NATUROPATH MIGHT RECOMMEND: Aim for around 450mg of mixed tocopherols.

FOOD SOURCES INCLUDE: Eggs; asparagus; peas; cucumber; millet; almonds; hazelnuts; sunflower seeds.

ZINC

Zinc is a very important mineral for the synthesis and metabolism of hormones. Zinc is involved in the synthesis of oestrogen and progesterone and transporting them around the body. Zinc is also used in egg production, ovulation and fertilisation. It may reduce inflammation, stimulate the immune system and is an antioxidant.

WHO MIGHT NEED IT? Zinc is recommended for vegans, vegetarians and women wanting to conceive. Zinc is essential for anybody currently taking or having recently used the oral contraceptive pill, which may increase copper and deplete zinc in the body. Conditions zinc is beneficial for include: PMS; period pain; endometriosis; PCOS; pelvic inflammatory disease; poor immunity (recurrent colds); cold sores; poor wound healing; acne; dermatitis; anxiety.

WHAT TO LOOK FOR: Zinc citrate and zinc picolinate are the most absorbable forms of zinc. Forms to avoid include zinc oxide and zinc sulphate as they do not absorb well in the body. Depending on dose, it is also best not to take zinc along with calcium and iron supplements as, depending on the dose of each nutrient, they may compete with each other for absorption. Check with your prescribing practitioner about whether this applies to you.

DAILY DOSAGE YOUR NATUROPATH MIGHT RECOMMEND: PMS: 50mg; Period pain: 20–30mg; Endometriosis: 60mg; PCOS: 30–60mg

FOOD SOURCES INCLUDE: Oysters; beef; shellfish; sesame seeds; pine nuts; cashews; pecans; buckwheat; legumes; pepitas (pumpkin seeds); sunflower seeds.

FOOTNOTES

1. Thaddeus T. Schug, Anne F. Johnson, Linda S. Birnbaum, Theo Colborn, Louis J. Guillette, Jr., David P. Crews, Terry Collins, Ana M. Soto, Frederick S. vom Saal, John A. McLachlan, Carlos Sonnenschein, Jerrold J. Heindel; Minireview: Endocrine Disruptors: Past Lessons and Future Directions, *Molecular Endocrinology*, Volume 30, Issue 8, 1 August 2016, Pages 833-847

2. Chinedum Onyenekwe Charles, Chukwudi Ezeani Michael, Ndidiamaka A Udeogu, Daniel C Anyiam, Samuel U Meludu, Okwudiri Nnadozie. Effect of Pre and Post Academic Examination Stress on Serum Level of Cortisol and Progesterone Circulation amongst Students of Nnamdi Azikiwe University Nnewi Campus Anambra State, Nigeria. *International Journal of TROPICAL DISEASE & Health*. 2014 Jan; 4(1): 62-69.

3. 'Foods that fight inflammation', *Harvard Health Publications*, June 2014; updated August 2017. **www.health.harvard.edu/staying-healthy/foods-that-fight-inflammation**

4. Ari Shechter and Diane B. Boivin, Sleep, Hormones, and Circadian Rhythms throughout the Menstrual Cycle in Healthy Women and Women with Premenstrual Dysphoric Disorder, *International Journal of Endocrinology*, vol. 2010, Article ID 259345, 17 pages, 2010. doi:10.1155/2010/259345 **and** Massimiliano de Zambotti, Adrian R. Willoughby, Stephanie A. Sassoon, Ian M. Colrain, Fiona C. Baker; Menstrual Cycle-Related Variation in Physiological Sleep in Women in the Early Menopausal Transition, *The Journal of Clinical Endocrinology & Metabolism*, Volume 100, Issue 8, 1 August 2015, Pages 2918–2926

5. M. Palmery, A. Saraceno, A. Vaiarelli, G. Carlomagno. Oral contraceptives and changes in nutritional requirements. *European Review for Medical and Pharmacological Sciences*, 2013, Vol. 17 - N. 13 Pages 1804-1813

6. Rose E. Frisch, *Female Fertility and the Body Fat Connection*, The University of Chicago Press, April 2002.

7. Rossi BV, Berry KF, Hornstein MD, Cramer DW, Ehrlich S, Missmer SA. Effect of Alcohol Consumption on In Vitro Fertilization. *Obstetrics and gynecology*. 2011;117(1):136-142.

8. Buck Louis GM, Sapra KJ, Schisterman EF, Lynch CD, Maisog JM, Grantz KL, Sundaram R. Lifestyle and pregnancy loss in a contemporary cohort of women recruited prior to conception, LIFE Study. *Fertility and Sterility* 2016;106(1):180-188. PMID: 27016456. A summary of the conclusions is available at **www.nih.gov/news-events/news-releases/couples-pre-pregnancy-caffeine-consumption-linked-miscarriage-risk**

9. Chavaro 2012. European Society of Human Reproduction and Embryology. A high intake of certain dietary fats associated with lower live birth rates in IVF. *ScienceDaily*. 3 July 2012. **www.sciencedaily.com/releases/2012/07/120703120655.htm**

10. MJ Ceko, K Hummitzsch, N Hatzirodos, WM Bonner, JB Aitken, DL Russell, M Lane, RJ Rodgers and HH Harris; X-Ray fluorescence imaging and other analyses identify selenium and GPX1 as important in female reproductive function. *Metallomics*. 2015, 7, 71-82

11. **www.foodstandards.gov.au/consumer/generalissues/hormonalgrowth/**

12. **www.foodstandards.gov.au/consumer/chemicals/bpa/**

13. Mnif W, Hassine AIH, Bouaziz A, Bartegi A, Thomas O, Roig B. Effect of Endocrine Disruptor Pesticides: A Review. *International Journal of Environmental Research and Public Health*. 2011; 8(6):2265-2303.

14. **www.choice.com.au/food-and-drink/food-warnings-and-safety/plastic/articles/bpa-in-canned-foods**

15. Harvey, Paul J; Handley, Heather K; Taylor, Mark. Widespread copper and lead contamination of household drinking water, New South Wales, Australia. *Environmental Research* (August, 2016).

16. **ntrs.nasa.gov/archive/nasa/casi.ntrs.nasa.gov/19930073077.pdf**

17. Wycliffe Wanzala, Ahmed Hassanali, Wolfgang Richard Mukabana, and Willem Takken, Repellent Activities of Essential Oils of Some Plants Used Traditionally to Control the Brown

Ear Tick, *Rhipicephalus appendiculatus. Journal of Parasitology Research*, vol. 2014, Article ID 434506, 10 pages, 2014.

18. Diamanti-Kandarakis E, Bourguignon J-P, Giudice LC, et al. Endocrine-Disrupting Chemicals: An Endocrine Society Scientific Statement. *Endocrine Reviews*. 2009; 30(4): 293-342.

19. Schlumpf M, Cotton B, Conscience M, Haller V, Steinmann B, Lichtensteiger W. In vitro and in vivo estrogenicity of UV screens. *Environmental Health Perspectives*. 2001; 109(3): 239-244.

20. Dinwiddie MT, Terry PD, Chen J. Recent Evidence Regarding Triclosan and Cancer Risk. *International Journal of Environmental Research and Public Health*. 2014;11(2):2209-2217 **and** Yuan M, Bai M-Z, Huang X-F, et al. Preimplantation Exposure to Bisphenol A and Triclosan May Lead to Implantation Failure in Humans. *BioMed Research International*. 2015; 2015:184845.

21. Petersen AB, Wulf HC, Gniadecki R, Gajkowska B; Dihydroxyacetone, the active browning ingredient in sunless tanning lotions, induces DNA damage, cell-cycle block and apoptosis in cultured HaCaT keratinocytes, *Mutation Research*, 2004 Jun 13; 560(2): 173-86.

22. Ferreira RC, Halpern G, Figueira Rde C, Braga DP, et al.; Physical activity, obesity and eating habits can influence assisted reproduction outcomes. *Women's Health* [Lond Engl] 2010. 6: 517-524.

23. Guseman, Emily & Zack, E & Battaglini, Claudio & Viru, Mehis & Viru, A & Hackney, Anthony. (2008). Exercise and circulating Cortisol levels: The intensity threshold effect. *Journal of endocrinological investigation*. 31. 587-91.

24. Taheri S, Lin L, Austin D, Young T, Mignot E. Short Sleep Duration Is Associated with Reduced Leptin, Elevated Ghrelin, and Increased Body Mass Index. Froguel P, ed. *PLoS Medicine*. 2004; 1(3): e62.

25. Lattimer JM, Haub MD. Effects of Dietary Fiber and Its Components on Metabolic Health. *Nutrients*. 2010; 2(12): 1266-1289. **and** Fuhrman BJ, Feigelson HS, Flores R, et al. Associations of the Fecal Microbiome With Urinary Estrogens and Estrogen Metabolites in Postmenopausal Women. *The Journal of Clinical Endocrinology and Metabolism*. 2014; 99(12): 4632-4640.

26. USDA. 2016. *Dairy 2014,* Dairy Cattle Management Practices in the United States, 2014, USDA–APHIS–VS–CEAH–NAHMS. Fort Collins, CO #692.0216

27. Malekinejad H, Rezabakhsh A. Hormones in Dairy Foods and Their Impact on Public Health - A Narrative Review Article. *Iranian Journal of Public Health*. 2015; 44(6): 742-758.

28. J.E. Chavarro, J.W. Rich-Edwards, B. Rosner, W.C. Willett; A prospective study of dairy foods intake and anovulatory infertility, *Human Reproduction*, Volume 22, Issue 5, 1 May 2007, Pages 1340–1347 **and** Rajaeieh G, Marasi M, Shahshahan Z, Hassanbeigi F, Safavi SM. The Relationship between Intake of Dairy Products and Polycystic Ovary Syndrome in Women Who Referred to Isfahan University of Medical Science Clinics in 2013. *International Journal of Preventive Medicine*. 2014; 5(6): 687-694.

29. Jianqin et al. 2016 'Effects of milk containing only A2 beta casein versus milk containing both A1 and A2 beta casein proteins on gastrointestinal physiology, symptoms of discomfort, and cognitive behavior of people with self-reported intolerance to traditional cows' milk'. *Nutrition Journal*. 2016 Apr 2; 15:35

30. Kratz, M.; Baars, T.; Guyenet, S. The relationship between high-fat dairy consumption and obesity, cardiovascular, and metabolic disease. *Eur. J. Nutr.* 2013, 52, 1–24 **and** Dairy consumption in association with weight change and risk of becoming overweight or obese in middle-aged and older women: a prospective cohort study. *American Journal of Clinical Nutrition*, 2016 103: 4 979-988

31. Swithers SE, Ogden SB, Davidson TL. Fat substitutes promote weight gain in rats consuming high-fat diets. *Behavioral neuroscience*. 2011; 125(4): 512-518.

32. Minihane AM, Vinoy S, Russell WR, et al. Low-grade inflammation, diet composition and health: current research evidence and its translation. *The British Journal of Nutrition*. 2015;114(7):999-1012 **and** Kevin L Fritsche, The Science of Fatty Acids and Inflammation. *Advances in Nutrition* May 2015 *Adv Nutr* vol. 6: 293S-301S, 2015.

33. Arentz S, Abbott JA, Smith CA and Bensoussan A. Herbal medicine for the management of polycystic ovary syndrome (PCOS) and associated oligo/amenorrhoea and hyperandrogenism; a review of the laboratory evidence for effects with corroborative clinical findings. *BMC Complementary and Alternative Medicine:* The official journal of the International Society for Complementary Medicine Research (ISCMR) 2014, 14: 511.

34. Grant P, Spearmint herbal tea has significant anti-androgen effects in polycystic ovarian syndrome. A randomized controlled trial. *Phytotherapy Research*. 2010 Feb; 24(2): 186-8 **and** Akdoğan M, Tamer MN, Cüre E, Cüre MC, Köroğlu BK, Delibaş N, Effect of spearmint (*Mentha spicata* Labiatae) teas on androgen levels in women with hirsutism, *Phytotherapy Research*. 2007 May; 21(5): 444-7.

35. Ibrahim NA, Shalaby AS, Farag RS, Elbaroty GS, Nofal SM, Hassan EM, Gynecological efficacy and chemical investigation of *Vitex agnus-castus* L. fruits growing in Egypt. *Natural Product Research*. 2008 Apr 15; 22(6): 537-46.

36. Bosma-den Boer MM, van Wetten M and Pruimboom L, Chronic inflammatory diseases are stimulated by current lifestyle: how diet, stress levels and medication prevent our body from recovering. *Nutrition & Metabolism*, 2012, 9: 32

37. Emanuele MA, WezemanF, and Emanuele, NV, Alcohol's Effects on Female Reproductive Function. National Institute on Alcohol Abuse and Alcoholism. June 2003. **pubs.niaaa.nih. gov/publications/arh26-4/274-281.htm**

38. Eggert J, Theobald H, Engfeldt P. Effects of alcohol consumption on female fertility during an 18-year period. *Fertility and Sterility*. 2004; 81(2): 379–83.

39. Lassi ZS, Imam AM, Dean SV and Bhutta ZA. Preconception care: caffeine, smoking, alcohol, drugs and other environmental chemical/radiation exposure. *Reproductive Health*. 2014. 11 (Suppl 3): S6.

40. Bailey RL, Mills JL, Yetley EA, et al. Unmetabolized serum folic acid and its relation to folic acid intake from diet and supplements in a nationally representative sample of adults aged ≥60 y in the United States. *The American Journal of Clinical Nutrition*. 2010; 92(2): 383-389 **and** Sweeney MR, Staines A, Daly L, et al. Persistent circulating unmetabolised folic acid in a setting of liberal voluntary folic acid fortification. Implications for further mandatory fortification? *BMC Public Health*. 2009; 9:295.

ADDITIONAL NOTES

Lignan (page 30): Higdon J, 'Lignans', Linus Pauling Institute, Oregon State University. **lpi.oregonstate. edu/mic/dietary-factors/phytochemicals/lignans**

Chocolate cravings (page 45): Ashley Mason and Elissa Epel, 'Craving Chocolate?: A Review of Individual Differences, Triggers, and Assessment of Food Cravings', in Avena N, *Hedonic Eating: How the Pleasurable Aspects of Food Can Affect Our Brains and Behavior*, Oxford University Press, May 2015.

Cramps (page 47): Minihane AM, Vinoy S, Russell WR, et al. Low-grade inflammation, diet composition and health: current research evidence and its translation. *The British Journal of Nutrition*. 2015; 114(7): 999-1012. doi:10.1017/S0007114515002093.

Antibacterial chemicals (page 90): US FDA bans chemicals in antibacterial hand soap over health concerns, *ABC News*, September 2016. **www.abc. net.au/news/2016-09-03/us-fda-bans-chemicals-in-anti-bacterial-hand-soap/7812182**

Stress (page 96): 'Estrogen Dominance' **www. drrind.com/therapies/estrogen-dominance**

Sleep and rest (page 99): 'How much sleep do you really need?' fact sheet from the Sleep Health Foundation. **www.sleephealthfoundation.org. au/public-information/fact-sheets-a-z/230-how-much-sleep-do-you-really-need.html**

Soy (page 123): Jefferson WN. Adult Ovarian Function Can Be Affected by High Levels of Soy. *The Journal of Nutrition*. 2010; 140(12): 2322S-2325S and Gu C, Pan H, Sun Z, Qin G. Effect of Soybean Variety on Anti-Nutritional Factors Content, and Growth Performance and Nutrients Metabolism in Rat. *International Journal of Molecular Sciences*. 2010; 11(3): 1048-1056.

Follicular phase (page 127): IMW Ebisch, CMG Thomas, WHM Peters, DDM Braat, RPM Steegers-Theunissen, The importance of folate, zinc and antioxidants in the pathogenesis and prevention of subfertility. *Human Reproduction Update,* Volume 13, Issue 2, 1 March 2007, Pages 163–174.

Added sugars (page 138): Ng SW, Slining MM, and Popkin BM. Use of caloric and noncaloric sweeteners in US consumer packaged foods, 2005-2009. *Journal of the Academy of Nutrition and Dietetics,* (2012) 112(11), 1828-1834.e1821-1826.

Honey (page 146): Eteraf-Oskouei T, Najafi M. Traditional and Modern Uses of Natural Honey in Human Diseases: A Review. *Iranian Journal of Basic Medical Sciences.* 2013; 16(6): 731-742; Carter DA, Blair SE, Cokcetin NN, et al. Therapeutic Manuka Honey: No Longer So Alternative. Frontiers in Microbiology. 2016; 7: 569; Mandal MD, Mandal S, Honey: its medicinal property and antibacterial activity. *Asian Pacific Journal of Tropical Biomedicine.* 2011;1(2):154-160.

Supplements (pages 232–239): R Rago, I Marcucci, G Leto, L Caponecchia, P Salacone, P Bonanni, C Fiori, G Sorrenti, A Sebastianelli, Effect of Myo-Inositol and Alpha-Lipoic Acid on Oocyte Quality in Polycystic Ovary Syndrome Non-Obese Women Undergoing in Vitro Fertilization: A Pilot Study. *Journal of Biological Regulation of Homeostatic Agents* 29 (4), 913-923. Oct-Dec 2015; Umesh Masharani, Christine Gjerde, Joseph L. Evans, Jack F. Youngren, Ira D. Goldfine, Effects of Controlled-Release Alpha Lipoic Acid in Lean, Nondiabetic Patients with Polycystic Ovary Syndrome. *Journal of Diabetes Science and Technology,* Vol 4, Issue 2, pp. 359 - 364; Bennett M, Vitamin B12 deficiency, infertility and recurrent fetal loss, *Journal of Reproductive Medicine.* 2001 Mar; 46(3): 209-12; Mgongo FO, Gombe S, Ogaa JS, The influence of cobalt/vitamin B12 deficiency as a 'stressor' affecting adrenal cortex and ovarian activities in goats. *Reproduction, Nutrition, Development,* 1984; 24(6): 845-54; Maurizio Nordio and Sabrina Basciani, Treatment with Myo-Inositol and Selenium Ensures Euthyroidism in Patients with Autoimmune Thyroiditis, *International Journal of Endocrinology,* vol. 2017, Article ID 2549491, 6 pages, 2017.

FURTHER READING:

Trickey, Ruth, *Women, Hormones and the Menstrual Cycle,* Trickey Enterprises (Victoria) Pty Limited, 2011

Harvey, Shannon, *The Whole Health Life,* Whole Health Life Publishing, 2016

Naish, Francesca, *Natural Fertility,* Milner Health Series, Sally Milner Publishing, first published 1991, Fourth Edition 2012

Collins, Gretchen Garbe, & Rossi, Brooke V., The impact of lifestyle modifications, diet, and vitamin supplementation on natural fertility, *Fertility Research and Practice,* 2015 1:11 **doi.org/10.1186/s40738-015-0003-4**

www.lowtoxlife.com

www.scientificamerican.com/article/toxins-all-around-us/

State of the science of endocrine disrupting chemicals (2012): **www.who.int/ceh/publications/endocrine/en/**

National Institute of Environmental Health Sciences: *Endocrine Disruptors.* **www.niehs.nih.gov/health/topics/agents/endocrine/**

Fertility Society of Australia fact sheet: *The role of exercise in improving fertility, quality of life and emotional well-being.* yourfertility.org.au/The-role-of-exercise-in-improving-fertility.pdf

Dr Sara Gottfried MD: *15 reasons to rethink red meat.* www.saragottfriedmd.com/15-reasons-to-rethink-red-meat/

US Food and Drug Administration (2004, November): *How to Understand and Use the Nutrition Facts Label.* www.fda.gov/food/ingredientspackaginglabeling/labelingnutrition/ucm274593.htm

INDEX

RECIPE INDEX

ACKNOWLEDGMENTS

Belinda: I would like to thank Ainsley for her amazing contributions to this book: when we first began, I could never have imagined that she would be so talented! Thank you also to the generous people who reviewed my words and gave invaluable feedback, including Dr Natasha Andreadis, Emma Sutherland, Alexx Stuart, Libby Babet and Dr Brad McEwen.

A big thank you to my beautiful family and friends for supporting me and believing in me; and a final thank you to my mentor, supporter and inspiration for all things naturopathic, Amanda Haberecht — thank you!

Ainsley: Thank you Belinda; this book would not exist without your outstanding expertise, experience, knowledge and passion.

Thank you to my very dear friend Lara Hutton, who came to my rescue with her marvellous props. Thank you to Studio Enti for your beautiful and inspiring ceramics. Also thanks to Zakkia Homewares.

Thank you to my girlfriends who road-tested my recipes with their families, providing essential and welcome feedback. And finally a big thanks to my gorgeous girls for their modelling help and to my husband, Matthew, for your endless support.

We would also love to thank our graphic designer, Lucille Grant, who went above and beyond to bring this beautiful book to life. Thank you also for introducing us to each other in the first place.

Thank you to our fantastic agent Pippa Masson at Curtis Brown and the fabulous team at Murdoch Books: we couldn't have done it without your support and guidance.

Published in 2018 by Murdoch Books, an imprint of Allen & Unwin

Murdoch Books Australia
83 Alexander Street, Crows Nest NSW 2065
Phone: +61 (0)2 8425 0100
murdochbooks.com.au
info@murdochbooks.com.au

Murdoch Books UK
Ormond House, 26–27 Boswell Street,
London, WC1N 3JZ
Phone: +44 (0) 20 8785 5995
murdochbooks.co.uk
info@murdochbooks.co.uk

For Corporate Orders & Custom Publishing contact our business
development team at salesenquiries@murdochbooks.com.au

Publisher: Corinne Roberts
Design Manager: Madeleine Kane
Editor: Melody Lord
Designer: Lucille Grant
Recipes, styling, photography and illustrations: Ainsley Johnstone
Production Manager: Lou Playfair

ISBN 978 1 74336 937 1 Australia
ISBN 978 1 74336 938 8 UK
A cataloguing-in-publication entry is available from the catalogue
of the National Library of Australia at nla.gov.au
A catalogue record for this book is available from the British Library

Colour reproduction by Splitting Image Colour Studio Pty Ltd, Clayton, Victoria
Printed by 1010 Printing, China

DISCLAIMER: The purchaser of this book understands that the information contained within is not
intended to replace one-to-one medical advice. It is understood that you will seek full medical clearance
by a licensed physician before making any changes mentioned in this book. The author and publisher
claim no responsibility to any person or entity for any liability, loss or damage caused or alleged to be
caused directly or indirectly as a result of the use, application or interpretation of the material in this book.

TABLESPOON MEASURES: We have used Australian 20 ml (4 teaspoon) tablespoon measures.
If you are using a smaller European 15 ml (3 teaspoon) tablespoon, add an extra teaspoon
of the ingredient for each tablespoon specified.